Open University Press
Celtic Court
22 Ballmoor
Buckingham
MK18 1XW

e-mail: enquiries@openup.co.uk
world wide web: http://www.openup.co.uk

and
325 Chestnut Street
Philadelphia, PA 19106, USA

First Published 2000

A catalogue record of this book is available from the British Library

ISBN   0 335 20364 7 (pb)   0 335 20365 5 (hb)

Library of Congress Cataloging-in-Publication Data
Gender inequalities in health/edited by Ellen Annandale and Kate
   Hunt.
      p. cm.
   Includes bibliographical references and index.
   ISBN 0-335-20365-5 (hbk.). – ISBN 0-335-20364-7 (pbk.)
   1. Health – Sex differences.   2. Medical care – Utilization – Sex
differences.   3. Sex discrimination in medicine.   I. Annandale,
Ellen. II. Hunt, Kate, 1959– .
RA564.B5.G4653   1999
362.1–dc21   99–30442
                                                              CIP

Typeset by Graphicraft Limited, Hong Kong
Printed in Great Britain by Biddles Ltd, Guildford and King's Lynn

Contents

Notes on contributors

Ellen Annandale is Senior Lecturer in Sociology at Leicester University. She is particularly interested in the relationship between the sociology of gender, feminist theory and research on gender, health and illness, and is currently writing *Feminist Theory and the Sociology of Health and Illness* (forthcoming). She is the author of *The Sociology of Health and Medicine* (1998).

Sara Arber is Professor and Head of the Department of Sociology at the University of Surrey. She is currently conducting research with Helen Cooper on older people and health inequalities, and on social support and health for the Health Education Authority. She is co-author with Jay Ginn of *Connecting Gender and Ageing* (Open University Press 1995).

Mick Carpenter is Reader in the Department of Social Policy and Social Work, and Co-Director of the Centre for Research in Health, Medicine and Society, at Warwick University. He has broad research interests in health policy, with inequalities as a central theme. He has acted as a policy adviser to a number of organizations, including the British public service union Unison. Recent publications include *Normality is Hard Work: Trade Unions and the Politics of Community Care* (1994).

Laurent Chenet is a population scientist at the London School of Hygiene and Tropical Medicine who specializes in developed countries' demography. His areas of research interest include the demography of countries in transition, socio-economic and sex differentials in mortality, and the impact of health policy. He is currently conducting research on Russia, the Ukraine and Lithuania.

Helen Cooper is a postgraduate student in the Department of Sociology at the University of Surrey, where she is investigating gender and ethnic differences in health using the Health Survey for England. Her work examines health inequalities across the lifecourse. With Sara Arber she has focused on the health of older adults and children.

Hilary Graham is Professor of Social Policy at Lancaster University. Her research and publications have focused on women's experiences of caring in poverty and how health related behaviours, including diet and smoking, are shaped by these experiences. The implications of increasing poverty and income inequalities in the UK for public health strategies has also been a theme of her work.

Keleigh Groves is currently undertaking a PhD on benefit fraud at the University of Leeds. Her research seeks to relate the meanings that people offer for their fraudulent action to a theoretical framework that acknowledges both social structure and creative human agency. This research is funded by a three-year Economic and Social Research Council (ESRC) research studentship.

Kate Hunt is a Senior Research Scientist at the Medical Research Council's Social and Public Health Sciences Unit at Glasgow University. She is a social scientist whose main interests are in gender and health, and the social construction of gender. Other current research includes inequalities in health (by social class and ethnicity as well as gender), and lay perceptions of inheritance and their influence on health related behaviours.

Jennie Popay is Professor of Sociology and Community Health and Director of the Public Health Research and Resource Centre at the University of Salford. She is also Associate Director of Research and Development for the Department of Health funded National Primary Care Research and Development Centre, and a non-executive board member of the Mancunian Community Health NHS Trust. She is a social scientist whose work has focused on the social patterning of health and illness, particularly gender inequalities; lay knowledge about health, illness and health care, family and child health; and health and social service policy analysis.

Ingrid Waldron is Professor of Biology and Donna and Larry Shelley Term Professor of Women's Studies at the University of Pennsylvania. She studies gender differences in health related behaviour and mortality, with a particular interest in recent trends in the USA. She also studies the effects of employment, marriage and parental status on women's health.

Preface

An influential body of research on gender inequalities in health has developed since the late 1960s. However, the combination of rapid social change in the lives of men and women in the last decades of the twentieth century, and an increased questioning of an oversimplified established wisdom about gender and health, makes a critical retrospective especially timely. The rationale for this collection lies both in recent developments in social theory which raise new questions about gender inequalities, and in the restructuring of gender related experiences which are likely to have widespread implications for the mental and physical health of men and women at the start of the twenty-first century. Each chapter questions some of the assumptions underlying the oversimplified orthodoxy and begins to identify ways to inject new energy into the debate.

All the chapters engage, to a greater or lesser degree, with current theoretical debates, some utilize published empirical data, while others involve new analyses of empirical data. Chapters 2 and 3 are orientated towards theoretical critiques of current research on gender and health (as is much of Chapter 1). The later chapters make more extensive use of empirical data, each focusing on different aspects of social change. Thus Hilary Graham (Chapter 4) is concerned with gender in the context of increasing socio-economic inequalities in Britain, Sara Arber and Helen Cooper (Chapter 5), also using data from Britain, focus on gender differences in health at three very different stages of the lifecourse, Ingrid Waldron (Chapter 6) draws on North American data for a detailed review of potential mechanisms underlying the changing pattern of mortality in the USA in the latter half of the twentieth century, and Laurent Chenet (Chapter 7) examines the impact on gender differences in health of the dramatic social changes following the collapse of former communist structures in eastern Europe during the late 1980s and 1990s. Like much research to date, the collection concentrates on gender and health in industrialized countries, with a particular focus on Britain, the USA and eastern Europe, and it focuses upon health status rather than wider questions such as the experience of health care.

In Chapter 1, Ellen Annandale and Kate Hunt outline general trends in research on gender and health since the 1970s when second wave feminism inspired an interest in the subject, highlighting methodological and theoretical concerns. They describe widespread social change, concentrating on changes in employment, educational qualifications, and the household and family, using Britain as a case study. They draw out three frameworks, the 'traditional', the 'transitional' and the emerging 'new', to summarize shifts in the theoretical and methodological approach to research on gender and health since the 1970s. The chapter argues in particular that research needs to be clearer than it has been to date about the nature of the social relations of gender as they impact upon the health of men and women.

In Chapter 2, Mick Carpenter also stresses the need for a critical reassessment of the theoretical foundations of this research and reviews issues arising out of the New Left and second wave feminism in the 1970s. He argues that problems with the 'second wave paradigm' need to be resolved, drawing on recent social and political theory, including postmodern analyses, work on masculinity, the sociology of the body and emotions, and puts forward eight 'realist' propositions for research on gender inequalities in health.

In Chapter 3, Jennie Popay and Keleigh Groves continue the critique of the 'grand narrative' of gender and health research on three counts: that research is affluence centred, ahistoric, and has neglected recent developments in social theory. They take up the criticisms of social role theory outlined in Chapter 1 by Annandale and Hunt. While Chapter 1 pointed to lack of clarity in terms of what 'gender' now means in the face of changes in society and theoretical critiques of gender from various forms of feminism and wider social theory, Popay and Groves also emphasize the need for greater attention to theory in the measurement of ill health in this area of research. There is, they suggest, much to be gained from more focused measures of health. They argue that qualitative research, and in particular narrative accounts, offers a means of exploring the relationship between structure and agency, illuminating the way in which men's and women's lives and health are differentially moulded and experienced.

In Chapter 4, Hilary Graham's focus is upon the consequences of rapid economic and social change for inequalities in health among men and women. Using UK data, she describes socio-economic inequalities in health, the factors which contribute to these health differences, and the ways in which they cluster together and accumulate through the lifecourse. She goes on to describe changing patterns of inequalities in wealth. She argues that little is known about the ways in which gender (and other axes of inequality such as ethnicity) mediate exposure to the influences underlying inequalities in health. Yet, she argues, social class 'expresses itself in a gendered form' and is 'written on the body'.

In Chapter 5, Sara Arber and Helen Cooper continue the theme of socio-economic inequalities in health. Using British data, they illustrate their contention that different factors should be considered at different stages in the lifecourse by analysing gradients in health among men and women at three distinct stages: childhood, the working ages and older adulthood. A lifecourse perspective, they argue, 'takes social change seriously and sees lives as dynamic and responsive to changed circumstances and opportunities'. Stages of the lifecourse are not merely distinguished by age but by the historical experiences that each generation has shared.

Chapters 6 and 7 move from a concern with morbidity to mortality. In Chapter 6, Ingrid Waldron takes a historical view of trends in mortality in the USA from 1950 to 1990. She examines trends in mortality sex ratios, analysing different causes of death and time periods separately, against several causal hypotheses to explain important recent changes in the patterns of gender and mortality. In Chapter 7, Laurent Chenet presents a series of analyses of trends in male and female mortality in a situation of extreme social change, namely the social turmoil following the collapse of communism in eastern Europe, focusing in detail on changes in mortality in Russia. He shows the very wide gender differences in mortality that are apparent in these countries, as men's mortality has worsened dramatically over a very short period of time. However, socio-economic differentials among women in Moscow are much greater than they are for men, in contrast to the patterns seen in much of the western world.

As it becomes increasingly widely accepted that the established wisdom 'women get sicker but men die quicker', which was based on research on gender and health from the 1970s, is an oversimplification, researchers in the field are increasingly striving to be more sensitive to the complexities of individuals' lives and more reflexive about the methodological premises that frame their research. While there are other issues that need to be addressed in this respect, such as the significance of ethnicity for gender differences in health, which are hinted at but not explored in detail here, we hope that the chapters in this book will feed into this debate and contribute to the resolution of the problems and challenges that this complexity presents for future for research.

Acknowledgements

The enthusiasm and motivation for initiating this book derives from discussions over a number of years with colleagues who share an interest in gender and health issues. We would like to thank all of these people, both colleagues in our own institutions and elsewhere, including of course all of the contributors to this collection. We would particularly like to acknowledge our debt to Judith Clark, Carol Emslie and Sally Macintyre with whom we have worked closely on some of the issues raised here. As ever the strictures of meeting deadlines have ramifications for others' lives, so thanks and love to Marc, Chloe and Lottie van Grieken, and to Nick James.

one

Gender inequalities in health: research at the crossroads

Ellen Annandale and
Kate Hunt

Introduction

Gender inequalities in health have been a major area of sociological research interest since the early 1970s. Rising to prominence on a wave of interest in the social relations of gender which challenged the empirical, theoretical and methodological core of sociology during the 1970s and early 1980s, the search for an explanation for differences in male and female morbidity and mortality, alongside interest in the relationship between variations in women's social circumstances and their health, has been a vital part of feminists' attempts to challenge the detrimental effects of patriarchy on women's health.

By the late 1970s a research orthodoxy had emerged, under the twin influences of liberal feminism's assimilationist agenda, which emphasized the health enhancing effects of access to social roles and statuses hitherto defined as male, and the radical feminist stress upon the primacy of gender over other statuses in the production of inequality (Annandale 1998a). This orthodoxy became a blueprint for research on gender differences in health which stressed entrenched inequalities in the experiences of women and men in the related spheres of paid and domestic work, and the consequences of these differences, for example for status and income. A distinction between sex (biology) and gender (the social) was essential to this tradition of research since it made clear that gender inequalities in health were in the most part socially produced, rather than biologically given. As such they could be ameliorated, even eradicated, through changes in the gender order. This orthodoxy, which generated an exciting and substantial body of research, prevailed largely unchallenged until the mid-1990s (although see e.g. Clarke 1983) when researchers began to express disquiet about its theoretical and conceptual foundations. Kandrack *et al.* (1994: 588), for example, wrote of a conceptual impasse and intellectual inertia in the field. They argued that 'our methods and theories seem incapable of taking us beyond rudimentary statistical findings' and called for a major conceptual leap forward.

The source of the conceptual impasse that Kandrack *et al.* (1994) and others have identified can be found in the very frameworks that laid the foundation for the field. Liberal feminism (with its emphasis upon the occupancy of social roles) and radical feminism (with its emphasis on gender as 'difference') have both been seriously questioned, in response to accelerated changes in society as an object of study, and in social theory as a basis of explanation. These developments have brought with them not only serious conceptual and methodological challenges, but also opportunities. Thus a new vibrancy is being injected into debates on gender inequalities in health as an emerging 'new agenda' challenges received wisdom.

However, the questions that are posed and the research agenda that they call forth are still in flux. We are led to ask, for example, to what extent should the ongoing social change in men and women's lives in the worlds of work, household and the family, leisure and consumption in western societies be understood in terms of greater equality or greater inequality? How are we to understand the new social relations of gender in this context – has patriarchy been superseded, or has it taken on new forms that no longer rely upon a binary division of gender? So far, these questions remain largely unaddressed in research on gender inequalities in health, despite receiving attention within wider sociology and feminism. Yet it is crucial that these questions are taken seriously within the field of health and illness, since a clear sense of what gender actually *means* as we reach the beginning of the twenty-first century is essential to research on inequalities in health status.

The aim of this chapter is to review the current status of research on gender inequalities in health with particular reference to theoretical and methodological concerns, drawing upon empirical data where appropriate. Some of these concerns are taken up in more detail in the chapters which follow. We begin by addressing the broad issue of social change in the lives of men and women in Britain, concentrating on changes in employment, educational achievement, and in the household and family since it has been argued that these are the most important areas in the 'transformation of gender' (Walby 1997) which has taken place since the 1970s. This section draws, among other sources, on Sylvia Walby's important book, in which she argues that 'fundamental transformations of gender relations in the contemporary Western World are affecting the economy and all forms of social relations' (Walby 1997: 1). This review of key aspects of social change is followed by a discussion of how these changes can be explained within a new social relations of gender. We then draw out three frameworks, which we label the 'traditional', the 'transitional' and the 'new', to summarize shifts in theoretical and empirical approaches to research on gender and health since the 1970s. Finally, we reflect on some of the complex epistemological and methodological issues which need to be addressed in order that research can ultimately move forward. The chapter concludes by highlighting, in summary form, the emerging 'new agenda' for research on gender inequalities in health 'at the crossroads'.

Social change in the lives of men and women

Gender related social change as reflected in patterns of employment, education, family and household structure, leisure and consumption at the societal level, and in the everyday experience of individual men and women, has been high on the policy agenda and a topic of widespread academic interest among social scientists since the mid-1980s. While many of these changes are massive in scope, they are complex and subject to diverse explanation. Walby's (1997: 1) argument about women's circumstances applies equally to men – contemporary lives are changing in complex ways, not simply for better or worse. In this section we outline social change related to employment, the household and the family, education, and the relationship between home and work. For each of these domains, we reflect critically upon existing linked research on gender and health status.

Changes in work and employment

The problematic history of the conceptualization of women within the sociology of work and employment is especially important to research on gender and health status which has had the link between employment and health at its core since its inception. Early research of the 1950s, 1960s and into the 1970s, operated on the premise that 'workers were men' (Crompton 1997). Other feminists pointed to the 'invisible woman' and raised concerns about taken-for-granted assumptions about the nature of men's and women's work (for example, that it was the physical conditions of work that counted for men, while for women it was friendship and social support that mattered). Alongside this, there was a propensity within research to see women's domestic roles and responsibilities as 'natural' and to interpret their labour market position as secondary to 'domestic commitments'. As Acker (1991: 170) has pointed out, the very concept of a 'job' is inextricably linked to gender as 'it assumes a particular organisation of domestic life and social production'.

In the field of health research, early work tended to draw upon male-only samples, or to assume that it was possible to extrapolate from men to women in a universalizing manner (Messing *et al.* 1993). Indeed, despite significant increases in women's labour force participation after the Second World War in the west, it was not until the 1970s that the health implications of their work became a centre of attention (Doyal 1994). By the mid- to late 1980s, the pendulum had swung resulting in a focus on women-only samples and work related differences in health among women (Sorensen and Verbrugge 1987). In addition, almost irrespective of the nature of the sample, assumptions continued to be made about which aspects of work were important to men and which to women (Hunt and Annandale 1993). There was then little truly comparative research. This again reflects the gendered assumptions that were woven into research on inequalities in health, stemming from the dominant ideologies of the time and pervasive gender differentiation in the labour market. Thus, even though gender related patterns of employment began to change during the 1970s, there was a lag before this was reflected in changed research paradigms. However, although research which explicitly concerns gender and work is still marked by a focus on female-only samples (and research on men's work and their health still tends not to have a *gender* focus), a new research vista has been opened up by rapid social change in the sphere of employment since the late 1980s. Here we briefly map some parameters of this change.

Crompton (1997) contends that an understanding of women and work needs to be placed in the context of the increasing economic polarization and material inequality that accompanies the marketization of society. With reference to contemporary Britain (although her observations are broadly relevant to other western societies), she extends Hutton's characterization of the '30:30:40' society to take account of the household and gender. In the '30:30:40' society, 'only around 40 per cent of the workforce enjoy tenured full-time employment or secure self-employment . . . , another 30 per cent are insecurely self-employed, involuntarily part-time, or casual workers; while the bottom 30 per cent, the marginalized, are idle or working for poverty wages' (Hutton 1995, quoted in Crompton 1997: 131). When gender is incorporated into this model, the picture as shown in Figure 1.1 emerges.

Figure 1.1   Employment and households in the 30:30:40 society

	30	30	40
Men	Unemployed	Insecure full time	Full time
Women	Unemployed	Insecure part time	Full time/part time

Source: Crompton 1997: 131

The model in Figure 1.1 encapsulates gender differences in forms of employment, where women predominate in part-time work as they are disproportionately affected by the casualization and flexibilization of the workforce. Thus, in 1997, fully 92 per cent of British men who were in paid work were employed full time, compared with just 57 per cent of women. Working patterns still vary much more according to parental status (particularly when there are pre-school age children in the household) among women than they do among men. Overall, more than eight in ten part-time employees were women in 1997 (Office for National Statistics (ONS) 1998) and nearly as many women now work part time as they do full time. Despite this gender difference, there has also been a major shift in male employment from permanent full-time work to part-time or temporary work (ONS 1998); indeed 11 per cent of men now work part time (Walby 1997). This has been contemporaneous with a decline in the total number of men in employment (which has disproportionately affected those lower down the social hierarchy), alongside a rise in the total number of women in employment.

The exact figure that is put on women's increased participation in employment depends on how work and employment are defined. Thus statistics which utilize a more inclusive definition tend to show figures for women that are closer to men. Labour Force Survey data from Britain show that 91 per cent of men of working age were economically active in 1971, compared to only 57 per cent of women.[1] Women's economic activity rates increased to 72 per cent by 1997, while men's rates declined to 85 per cent over the same period (ONS 1998). But as Walby (1997: 29–30) notes, at the household level, the decline in male employment should not be taken as precipitating female employment. This has been reflected in the growth of 'no-earner' households (see Graham, Chapter 4 in this volume). Indeed, income support systems within Britain may even inhibit women's paid employment. For example, when after six months' unemployment a woman's husband moves from an individually based insurance benefit to income support, which is means-tested at the household level, it is typically not worthwhile in financial terms for her to work. Ethnic variations are also important, with differences in labour force participation generally being larger among women than among men. While the highest economic activity levels are among 'white' men and women (86 per cent and 72 per cent, respectively), Pakistani/Bangladeshi women have particularly low economic activity rates (25 per cent) (Walby 1997: 61, see also ONS 1998: 28). Part-time work especially is lower among minority ethnic women than it is among the majority 'white' population.

Walby summarizes the shift in gender related employment patterns as follows:

> During the post-war period and especially in the last decade there have been very significant changes in the position of women in employment. Women are almost as likely as men to be employed; but almost all of this increase is in part-time work. There has been a significant narrowing of the wages gap between women and men who work full-time, but this does not extend to women who work part-time. There has been a major increase in the proportion of women in top jobs, but significant sex segregation in employment still remains.
>
> (Walby 1997: 36–7)

Gender segregation within the labour market is pervasive, although the actual jobs that are characterized as 'male' or 'female' may change over time (see Alvesson and Billing 1997, for example). Thus, at present the main employment sectors for women in Britain are 'public administration, education and health' and 'distribution, hotels and restaurants', and it is in these same sectors where most part-time female employees are found. Indeed, part-time work exceeds full-time work in the 'distribution, hotels, and restaurant sector' (ONS 1998). Although the manufacturing sector has significantly declined since the 1970s – from a 32 per cent share of employment in 1973 to 19 per cent in 1993, representing a decline from 7.8 to 4.6 million people (Office of Population Censuses and Surveys (OPCS) 1995) – it is still the sector in which most male employees work. Part-time work is relatively rare in manufacturing, especially for male employees (ONS 1998). While manufacturing continues to decline, the female dominated service sector is predicted to rise to 74 per cent (17.0 million people) by the year 2000 (OPCS 1995).

There is some evidence of reduction in gender differences within more specific occupational areas. Thus, using British census data from 1981 and 1991, Walby considers 15 'occupational orders' to demonstrate that while one gender still tends to predominate in most occupations, 'women have increased their participation in the upper occupational orders and reduced them in lower ones – the higher the order the more likely an increase in both the absolute and relative numbers of women' (Walby 1997: 35). There has been a 155 per cent increase in women in the 'highest' occupational order ('professional and related supporting management; senior national and local government managers') over the period, compared to a 33 per cent increase among men. Female 'gains' can also be seen among specific occupations. For example, the proportion of female solicitors holding practising certificates rose from 20 per cent in 1988 to 33 per cent in 1997 in England and Wales and the proportion of female barristers rose from 14 per cent in 1987 to 24 per cent in 1997 (ONS 1998). However, vertical segregation remains (Arber and Gilbert 1992): even where women have entered 'male' jobs, they tend to remain at the bottom of the ladder; and within 'female' jobs, men are over-represented at the more senior levels (Williams 1992). Some have suggested that the breakthrough of women into higher status occupations is little more than cosmetic (Savage 1992), and that even within the same job title, men and women may actually undertake quite different work, in different conditions and with a male power structure still essentially intact. It has also been argued that women have had the greatest success in 'infiltrating' those male jobs which are least attractive (in terms of working conditions, power and economic rewards) to men (see e.g. Legge's (1987) discussion of personnel management).

While the trends towards greater equality of men and women in the labour market are important in and of themselves, they are only markers for broader changes in labour market experience. An important theme in this regard is the emergence of new forms of *work environment*. For example, although definitional problems make it difficult to give accurate figures for 'homeworking', the 1991 British census indicated that 1.2 million people conduct paid work 'mainly from home' (Crompton 1997), undertaking work as wide ranging as clothing assembly, packing products, electrical assembling and craft knitting, and women typically predominate in lower level work (see e.g. Phizacklea and Wolkowitz 1995). Teleworking, itself a very diverse category, is becoming increasingly significant, and the electronic cottage is seen by many as the workplace of the future (Crompton 1997). When compared to the traditional workplace, homeworking disperses the workforce across both place and time. Of equal interest in terms of new work environments is the emergence of Call Centres which, in contrast, aggregate large numbers of people into one place in a manner reminiscent of the heyday of factory manufacturing. It has been estimated that two-thirds of all Call Centre workers are women and that Call Centres will account for one in every fifty jobs by the year 2000 (Stanford 1999). As research on gender and health has a longstanding concern with 'combining' domestic and paid work and, more recently, with the similarities in conditions and the experience of work in each sphere for men and women, the advent of widespread homeworking is likely to be extremely interesting in relation to health given the collapse, or blurring, of distinctions between the 'home' and 'work' environments. Women or men who undertake homeworking will thus be subject to the conditions of their 'home' environment through both their unpaid 'domestic' work (see Bartley *et al.* 1992) and paid work. For those living in the least affluent conditions, this may present a double jeopardy to their health and, if more women undertake the least attractive 'homeworking' jobs, a yet more complex interaction between gender and socio-economic status may unfold.

Whether we examine the gender balance in more traditional or newly emerging employment sectors, it is crucial that we look beyond tabulations of gender similarities and differences in the terms, conditions and experiences of work. Since the late 1980s, research on gender, work and employment has turned its attention increasingly towards the ways in which different kinds of gender identities are *actively constructed* in the workplace (see e.g. Pringle 1988; Crompton 1997), and the supposed gender neutrality of conventional organizational theory has been subject to a fierce critique (see e.g. Acker 1991; Mills and Tancred 1992; Witz and Savage 1992; Halford *et al.* 1997). 'Appropriate' performances of gender may be achieved through diverse means, from male and female codes of dress, sexual harassment, or the predominance of a masculine culture of sexuality (see e.g. Collinson and Collinson 1990), and restriction of knowledge and opportunities by the exclusion of one gender. Gender relations therefore emerge and are subject to ongoing negotiation within the workplace (be this the factory or office, the Call Centre, the homework environment or the domestic workplace). There has been little research on the health implications of this *process* within research on gender inequalities in health, which has tended to utilize rather static notions of social roles and experiences in relation to work and health. In Chapter 3, Popay and Groves are also critical of this tendency within existing research and point to the ways in which the narrative method can move research forward.

Although paid work has been a major interest within research on gender inequalities in health in and of itself, it has also been of central concern because occupation has often been the basis of assigning a position in a *socio-economic hierarchy*. The theoretical power of socio-economic status as a concept derives from its holistic character as it draws together several facets of an individual's life under one umbrella term. Measures of socio-economic status such as education and occupation thus 'stand for' a complex conceptualization of a person's economic power and social standing. The difficulties that this poses are intensified by conceptual confusion over what social class/socio-economic status actually stands for theoretically, notably as it intersects with gender (Crompton and Mann 1994).

Occupation and, to a lesser extent, education are the most often used *indicators* of socio-economic status in research on health, although the use of occupational social class has been highly contested. The strands of this debate are both empirical and theoretical. Empirically, the British Registrar General's classification of occupations is based on a male occupational structure and, because of the entrenched gender segregation discussed above, fails to adequately discriminate between women's jobs (which cluster in social class III non-manual – secretaries, sales assistants, clerical workers, for example). As a consequence, socio-economic gradients in health tend to be shallower among women than among men (Pugh and Moser 1990; Pugh *et al.* 1991; Koskinen and Martelin 1994), although gradients are less too by some other measures (Macintyre and Hunt 1997). Second, women's occupations often do not 'match' their educational achievements due to movement out of the labour force, and discrimination within employment inhibiting the promotion of women. As the structure of employment changes, many of these problems may also concern men. One 'solution' to these problems of 'women's social class' has been to move from an individually to a household based measure of social class, typically relying on the male 'head of household' (Goldthorpe 1983). Objections to this have long been raised on the grounds that women are subsumed under men and that such household based measures are assumed to stand equally for all household members, when in fact access to household assets (while formally communal) may be highly gendered (Payne 1991). The conclusion is obvious, but crucially important for the study of gender inequalities in health – one is simply not comparing like with like (Payne 1991; Hunt and Macintyre in press).

These technical debates on the operationalization of socio-economic status have pervaded discussion of gender inequalities in health status, although in empirical research they have been more commonly raised in the context of differences among women than in comparative research including men. In a time of rapid and complex social change in the lives of men and women which is generating new lines of economic inequality (see Graham, Chapter 4), it is crucially important to capture gender differences in socio-economic status in a way that permits valid gender comparative research. Certainly the evidence that does exist to date suggests that systematically comparing inequalities among men and among women, and trying to account for similarities and differences (looking at different health outcomes, different age groups, and so on), could provide major clues to the aetiology of ill health, and inequalities, in both men and women (Macintyre and Hunt 1997; Hunt and Macintyre in press).

To summarize this section of the chapter which has been concerned with changes in work and employment: since around the late 1970s there has been a complex restructuring of employment which is likely to have differential impacts upon different 'groups' of women and men, generating new forms of equality and inequality. While some female 'gains' are apparent, 'there can be no sweeping statement about women catching up with men', nor does the pattern of gender related change fit neatly into a conceptualization of 'gender as opposition' (Walby 1997: 47). One of the most notable new divisions that is apparent is between different *age groups*. As Walby notes,

> to a significant extent women are polarising between those, typically younger, educated and employed, who engage in new patterns of gender relations somewhat convergent with those of men, and those, particularly disadvantaged women, typically older and less educated, who built their life trajectories around patterns of private patriarchy [i.e. subordination within the domestic realm]. These new patterns are intertwined with diversities and inequalities generated by social divisions including class, ethnicity and region.
>
> (Walby 1997: 2)

There is a need for research on health status to take these more recent patterns of inequality between women into account. But equally, there is a need to consider new forms of equality and inequality between men and women. There is a tendency even today within wider commentaries on gender and social change to foreground women's experience, leaving men's experience as a largely unarticulated backdrop. As noted earlier, this continues a long legacy of research on work and health in which the empirical spotlight is upon *either* women *or* men. However, in common with the wider field of gender and health inequalities, research which considers the relationship between employment and health is addressing an increasingly sophisticated agenda, in response to the increasing diversity and complexity of men's and women's lives. Some of the most important of these are summarized in Figure 1.2.

Figure 1.2 highlights moves towards a more *inclusive* research agenda around paid work, gender and health. However, at the moment, this movement is both rather piecemeal and inhibited by the quality of existing large scale statistical data sets which often contain limited or crude measures of paid work circumstances and health status, which make sensitive operationalization very difficult. Quantitative research on employment and health which seeks to use gender comparative samples

Figure 1.2   The changing focus of research on gender, paid work and health

The move away from	Towards
1 Male-only and female-only samples	1 Gender comparative samples
2 Certain aspects of work relevant to men's and other aspects relevant to women's health	2 All aspects of work relevant in principle to men and to women
3 Limited focus on 'role occupancy' (e.g. in work or not), especially in women-only studies	3 Concern with wider dimensions of work experience (e.g. physical and psychosocial work conditions)
4 Concern with limited aspects of health	4 (a) Recognition that work may have differential effects on different dimensions of health; (b) a more holistic approach towards health
5 Men and women conceptualized as isolated individuals	5 Contextualized as part of wider social structures (e.g. household, workplace) that is a social relations of gender
6 Limited focus on specific 'role combinations' (e.g. in work and home)	6 Attention to (a) complexity of interacting roles and statuses; (b) people's experience of a role
7 Failure to look at the active construction of gender in various contexts	7 Consideration of gender as constituted and reconstituted within the workplace and its implications for health

is also constrained by the continuing extent of gender segregation. Except at the higher levels of aggregation (e.g. occupational orders), it remains difficult to find sufficiently large numbers of men and women doing the same jobs to undertake more sophisticated analyses that can take more sensitive account of other domains of men's and women's lives (see Emslie *et al.* 1999).

It is now widely recognized that paid employment in and of itself generally has a beneficial effect on health (with those in paid work tending to be in better health than those who are not) (Waldron *et al.* 1998). However, this finding is tempered by the specific terms and conditions of employment, and the relationship between paid work and other aspects of men's and women's lives. For this reason, we will suspend a more detailed consideration of empirical research until we have looked at recent changes in the domains of education, and the family and household.

Changes in education

Walby (1997) argues that, alongside women's movement into paid employment, education is at the leading edge of the shift from a domestic to a public gender regime. Education is also crucial in marking out new patterns of increased inequality between women. For example, it differentiates between those younger women who are formally educated to levels that meet, or even exceed, those of similar aged men, and older women who have until the 1990s been excluded from the labour market and had few educational opportunities earlier in life.

There is evidence that women have made more rapid gains than men in educational terms in the 1990s. In Britain, entry into further education has increased significantly for both men and women (ONS 1998), but the number of women undergraduates increased by over 115 per cent between 1975–6 and 1992–3, while that of men increased by only 35 per cent. Improvement in the advanced (A level) school examinations was also greater for women than for men between 1975 and 1985 (ONS 1998), and young women made up 53 per cent of those with two or more A level passes in 1993–4. The proportion of young women aged 17 who gained three or more A levels rose from 9 per cent in 1985–6 (compared to 10 per cent of men) to 16 per cent in 1993–4 (compared to 14 per cent for men). In 1995–6, at the lower level of national school examinations (grades A to C GCSE or SCE level), 51 per cent of women compared with only 41 per cent of men aged 16 in the UK achieved five or more passes (Walby 1997).

In the context of gender inequalities in health status, Arber (1997) has argued:

> it is timely to reassess the value of educational qualifications in the British context, especially among women, where it is acknowledged that occupational class is a less than ideal measure because of downgrading following childbirth. Educational qualifications are a major factor in obtaining many jobs and promotion within occupations.
>
> (Arber 1997: 775)

Thus Arber argues that educational qualifications are a more robust measure of socio-economic status than occupational social class since they are strongly related to occupational achievement, but also a stable measure for those who fail to reach or sustain a level of occupational achievement that is consistent with their qualifications (through illness or exit from the labour force to rear children, for example). Moreover, educational qualifications offer the potential for greater discrimination between both women and (with labour market exclusions increasing) men. In this respect, it should be noted that occupational social class has had more prominence in British studies of health inequalities than elsewhere.

Since the 'success' of women in education only dates from around the mid-1980s, there is still a marked female educational disadvantage among older age groups. Using the British National Vocational Qualifications (NVQ) classificatory scheme, there was very little difference between the qualification levels of men and women aged 16–24 in 1997–8. However, by age 25–34, men's qualifications exceeded those of women. In older age groups, differences are even more marked, with the number of women holding no qualifications at all far exceeding men (ONS 1998). This pattern of gender difference by educational achievement, whereby younger women are converging with men (i.e. a pattern of emerging equality), but where there are profound inequalities by age within women (and persistent, but less marked, inequalities by age within men), highlights the complex nature of gender inequalities at the beginning of the twenty-first century.

Of course, possession of qualifications does not translate simply into success in the public sphere of work, as noted earlier. Discrimination in recruitment and promotion, and work related experiences such as sexual harassment, persist because of direct and indirect male exclusionary practices (see e.g. Witz 1990; Crompton 1997). A greater openness to the actual constitution of gender relations in the workplace, as described above, should help us to look at not only the complex ways in which educational qualifications are, or are not, 'translated' into success in the workplace, and the role of gender as part of this, but also the impact of the positioning of men and women in various ways upon psychosocial health – perhaps, for example, through the experience of status incongruity between potential and current achievement.

Changes in the family and the household

There is an explicit association between the changes in employment and other aspects of people's lives. As Crompton notes (1997: 3), the rise in women's employment 'has been accompanied by a falling birth rate, a rise in single-parent households, and an increase in the divorce rate' while 'much of the expansion of women's employment has been in the area of "non-standard" jobs, and . . . women's continuing family responsibilities loom large as a reason for taking up and continuing this kind of paid work'. The trends in patterns of marriage, parenting and fertility and in women's greater inroads into paid employment are not merely coincidental. Equal employment opportunities and control over fertility through wider access to contraception and termination of pregnancy were two key foci of second wave feminism.

Following the 'baby boom' of the 1960s (when there were around 80 live births per 1000 women), fertility rates for women aged 15–44 declined until the late 1970s (at which point there was a slight increase). During the 1980s and 1990s, rates remained fairly stable at around 60 live births per 1000 women. These rates conceal considerable age variations including a marked shift towards later childbearing. In England and Wales, the mean age of mothers at childbirth rose from 24.4 years in 1977 to 26.8 years in 1997. Fertility rates for women in their 20s have been falling, while those for women in their 30s have been rising. In addition, there has been a rapid increase in the number of women who remain childless at the age of 45 (from 9 per cent of women born in 1946 in England and Wales to 15 per cent for those born just five years later in 1951). It is projected that as many as one in five women born in 1961 will remain childless (ONS 1998).

Alongside these changes in fertility patterns, there have been major changes in patterns of marriage and divorce. Most notably, the number of first marriages has declined rapidly since the early 1970s in the UK, while the number of divorces and remarriages has risen. Divorce rates vary markedly by age, with higher numbers concentrated in younger age groups (those under age 25 have experienced the biggest growth). Data for 1996–7 indicate that, overall, men are more likely to be married than women (62 per cent compared to 58 per cent) and also more likely to be single (28 per cent compared to 22 per cent). This reflects the greater propensity for women to be either widowed or divorced (12 per cent and 7 per cent, respectively) than men (4 per cent and 6 per cent). Changes in marriage patterns have been associated with a rise in cohabitation; more than one in five non-married adults in Britain were cohabiting during 1996–7. While most adults still live in a couple household, there are important gender differences. Women are more likely than men to live in a household without another adult, either as lone parents or as an elderly person. Lone parenthood is often associated with material deprivation (see Graham, Chapter 4) and with relatively poor health for men and women (see e.g. Popay and Jones 1990; Macran *et al.* 1996). (This summary is drawn from ONS 1998.)

These trends have potentially wide-ranging ramifications for the study of gender and health, especially when considered alongside changing patterns of work. As we stress throughout this chapter, such changes in the lives of research subjects require us to rethink the ways in which we conceptualize the research agenda. The use of marital status categories is one pertinent example of the problem of trying to take account of diversity of experience while using the normative understandings which are embedded in official statistics and social surveys. As Arber (1997) notes, research of the 1970s and 1980s tended to show that previously married people have the worst health (a finding that holds particularly for women); that married people have better health than single people; but that the marital advantage is more evident for men than for women. However, 'it may be that more recent changes in marriage patterns, particularly the increase in divorce, and growth in cohabitation has meant that [these] earlier relationships . . . no longer hold' (Arber 1997: 776). Furthermore, Graham (1993: 14) recounts the problems of relying on data which present people's lives through categories which give them 'clear, stable and singular identities'. Thus, one cannot be simultaneously married and single so 'it is women's [and men's] legal status that drives the classification, not the meanings [they] give to their personal relationships' (Graham 1993: 32). (Another illustration given by Graham is that, since cohabitation is usually defined in heterosexual terms, gay men and women are typically construed as outside marriage/cohabitation, which may be at variance with their experience, and a violation of their sense of self.) Yet far from being static, marriage and other relationship statuses are currently subject to significant change as 'more women [and also men] are experiencing periods of living alone, living with a partner, marrying, divorcing and becoming lone mothers [and fathers]'. Thus 'individual biographies remind us that the labels ascribed to women [and men] do not describe a permanent status' (Graham 1993: 40).

These conceptual points notwithstanding, one issue that has been central to research on gender, health and the household, has been the domestic division of labour. Interest in whether either 'housewives' or women in paid work are in better health has continued since the 1970s. Early work tended to concentrate on the simple occupancy of the 'housewife' or 'paid worker' role, with little attention to the nature and quality of each 'role'. This of course mirrors the way in which the paid work–health relationship was approached (see Figure 1.2). Women-only samples have been the norm and it is only since the late 1980s that researchers have begun to develop more sophisticated models in which paid work and domestic work in their complexity are addressed in an adequate manner with comparative attention to both women and men. This incipient shift in research attention makes it important that we look more generally at whether the domestic gender division of labour is changing alongside, or perhaps as a result of, changing patterns in men's and women's paid work.

Although this is a contentious area, there is some evidence that the amount of work that women undertake in the home has declined as they have entered paid employment in larger numbers. Looking at trends over the period 1975–87, Gershuny *et al.* (1994) reported that husbands of full-time employed women had increased their proportion of housework the most. However, decreases in gender differences in time spent in housework are equally likely to be a result of working women (especially those who work full time) reducing their hours, rather than men increasing theirs (Crompton 1997; Walby 1997). Consequently, while recent data suggest that both men and women who are in paid work spend less time on domestic chores than those who are not in paid work in Britain, there is still evidence that 'gender differences in time use appear to persist despite a variety of lifestyles in different families' (ONS 1998: 64). Thus if we consider the crude division of domestic tasks, among eight out of ten married and cohabiting heterosexual couples in 1994, it was still the woman who 'always or usually' did the washing and ironing, while for three-quarters it was still the man who 'always or usually' did repairs around the house. A larger percentage of couples reported that other 'tasks' were more equally shared (about 45 per cent described looking after sick family members, as 'about equal or both together' and the corresponding figure was 52 per cent for shopping for groceries), although the remaining couples reported that these tasks were more likely to be 'usually or always' undertaken by the woman (ONS 1998). However, data from the 1991 British Social Attitudes Survey point towards an interesting gap between these reported actions and prevailing attitudes. Thus, while 62 per cent of couples felt that household cleaning *should* be shared equally, only 27 per cent of couples actually reported that they did share (and it has been noted that reports of time spent on, or sharing, household activities are themselves quite subjective). At the very least, as Crompton (1997: 87) concludes from a review of existing research, 'although men do take on more domestic work as a consequence of their female partner's paid employment, . . . this increase does not equalise the amount of work carried out by men and women.'

Informal caring work has also typically been perceived as gendered. Data from the 1991 British Household Panel Survey show that 17 per cent of women and 12 per cent of men looked after or gave special help to people who were sick or disabled either within or outside the household (Walby 1997). Research from the 1990 General Household Survey (GHS) shows that there were 3.4 million adults in Britain who were *sole* carers for relatives, friends and neighbours who were sick, handicapped or elderly. Although gender differences in the sample are again relatively small – 17 per cent of women and 14 per cent of men are carers –

women are more likely to be sole carers than men (57 per cent versus 42 per cent) and to be involved in caring for more hours per week (Evandrou 1996).

On the optimistic side, perhaps as Gershuny *et al.* (1994) suggest, we are witnessing a process of 'lagged adaptation' as changes in the household begin to 'catch up' with the changing realities of men's and women's paid employment. Moreover, the incipient move towards a somewhat more equal division of labour in some households in western societies is occurring alongside a rise in the availability of domestic goods. By 1994, 89 per cent of British households had a washing machine, 85 per cent of households had central heating and 67 per cent had a microwave oven (equivalent figures for 1979 were 75, 55 and 30 per cent respectively: Walby 1997). While it is important to appreciate, as Graham argues in Chapter 4 (see also Graham 1993), that both absolute and relative deprivation has been widening within Britain over this period, and this is disproportionately affecting lone female parents, it is a salutary reminder that patterns of domestic inequality are significantly more marked in third world countries where domestic work is especially open ended. Doyal (1995: 31) points out that the 'rigours of domestic work are at their most severe' in the third world where women 'weave their patchwork of survival through the direct production of their own and their family's needs'.

The picture that we have presented here of the domain of the household and of the family is no more than a snapshot. The concerns that we have concentrated upon (marital status, fertility and lone parenthood, and the domestic division of labour) are those which have predominated in discussions of gender and health status. In many self-evident ways, this manner of conceptualizing life in the family and household is woefully inadequate. We have little sense, for example, of how the various 'roles' that we have highlighted, such as that of lone parent, part-time paid worker with low status and low wages, in a new relationship, actually combine to influence health. We have even less sense of individuals' actual *experience* of this and other real life situations and how they might compare to those of other men and women. Furthermore, we often take an 'atomized', rather than an integrated, view of these domains of life; looking separately at men's and women's positions within the occupational structure and at their 'family' circumstances, for example, may obscure some very gendered patterns. 'Achieving' a certain place within the labour market may bring more hard choices for women than for men. Certainly, there is evidence that when and whether women have children (or a partner) varies more by occupational position for women than it does for men (see e.g. Emslie *et al.* 1999).

Without these more complex understandings, there is little or no opportunity to explore any similarities by gender that might be embedded in different complex social circumstances (see also Popay and Groves, Chapter 3 in this collection). Additionally, there are whole swathes of 'domestic life' which remain largely untouched by existing mainstream research on gender and health. One example of this is domestic violence which is a public issue on a global scale (Doyal 1995). The World Development Report of 1993 indicates that 'rape and domestic violence together account for about five per cent of the total disease burden of women aged fifteen to 44 in developing countries and nineteen per cent in developed countries' (cited in Doyal 1995: 53). Marriage, cohabitation and other forms of intimate relationship then seem to offer a veritable cornucopia of unexplored benefits and losses for health much in the same way that we have described for paid work. Finally, in spite of the established finding of the 'marriage advantage' (referred to above), the balance sheet for men is even more obscure at the present time as gender related social changes pose new challenges to traditional patriarchal forms. A crucial question, which we take up in broader terms later in the chapter, is the significance of the changing world of employment for men (notably rising unemployment in lower social strata) and the emergence of what some social theorists have called 'new ways of living' in the personal sphere (Beck and Beck-Gernsheim 1995). Giddens (1992), for example, positions women as the prime movers in what he calls the developing 'democratisation of the personal sphere', by which he means the emergence of free and equal relations between people. Yet Pahl (1995) contends that men are ill equipped for the 'new world' of work today (i.e. for the loss of the 'provider role') and that their emotional reticence makes it difficult for them to adapt to changes in domestic circumstances.

Research on paid work, domestic work and health status

Lorber (1997) reminds us that

> jobs and families are complex variables with good and bad effects on the physical and mental health of women and men. Both are areas for social support, which is beneficial to health; both are sometimes hazardous environments with detrimental physical effects; both produce stress.

(Lorber 1997: 27)

In research terms, it is now appreciated that since neither 'women' nor 'work' are homogenous categories, large scale comparisons of women in the home and women in work are of little real use (Doyal 1994).

Rather, 'the key question is not whether paid work in general is good for all women, but rather what the conditions are under which specific types of work will be harmful or beneficial for particular women in particular circumstances' (Doyal 1994: 67; see also Waldron 1991). The same points pertain to men.

Understanding of the relationship between paid work, domestic work and health status has taken a series of important conceptual steps forward over a relatively short time period. The following six developments are key.

First, as noted above, research began with large scale comparisons between women who were in paid work and full-time 'housewives'. This research culminated in the general conclusion that *women in paid work tend to be in better health than those who are not* (Nathanson 1975).

Second, questions were then raised about possible *health selection effects* (that is, perhaps it is not so much that being full time in the home has a negative impact upon health, but that unhealthy people are being excluded from the workforce). However, subsequent analyses have generally confirmed that the better health of employed women does not simply reflect a 'healthy worker effect' (Arber 1997).

Third, research then began to *build a range of additional work and family related factors into analyses* (Nathanson 1980). For example, researchers considered if the protective effect of paid work upon health for women was mediated by whether it was full or part time, with many (though not all) researchers concluding that it is often part-time work that is associated with better health. They also looked at marital status (Kane 1994); the presence of children (of various ages) in the household (Arber *et al.* 1985; Verbrugge 1989); and socio-economic status (variously measured, see above). The conceptual framework that was employed was very much that of 'role relationships' with the emphasis squarely upon the basic occupancy of a role (see Figure 1.2).

Fourth, an influential set of basic hypotheses emerged which raised the question of whether the *occupancy of 'multiple roles'* was positive ('role accumulation', 'role enhancement') or negative ('role strain') for women's health. The general finding was that multiple role occupancy was good for health. Thus in the early 1980s, Verbrugge (1983: 26) concluded that 'there is no evidence that multiple roles harm women's health, or for that matter men's'. In a later article with Sorensen, she expressed her view that benefits can be additive, or they may be synergistic:

> when troubles arise in one role, the others may offer supports and buffers such as overt advice and empathy, a place to renew energy and self-esteem, and a means of locating people and resources to solve the problem. Multiple roles offer excuses; obligations in one

arena can be dropped by citing responsibilities in another. Being very busy with roles can make someone's feelings of worth and excitement bound upward.

(Sorenson and Verbrugge 1987: 244)

The multiple role framework continues to be influential today as researchers develop increasingly complex hypotheses about the beneficial and harmful health effects of various specific roles and role combinations. Thus, drawing upon longitudinal data (for 1968 and 1988) from the USA to explore three 'roles' (marriage, employment and parenthood), Waldron *et al.* (1998) have concluded that 'role substitution' is the most successful of a series of hypotheses in explaining women's physical health status. 'Role substitution' means that when two roles perform similar functions they substitute for each other. For example, the authors suggest that 'employment and marriage may substitute for each other as sources of income, health insurance, and social support' (Waldron *et al.* 1998: 218).

Fifth, although the underlying premise of this body of research has been that if women were in the same role positions as men, then there would be little or no difference in their health status, until the late 1980s there has been very little *gender comparative research* (as stressed throughout this chapter). In part this neglect has been theoretical: traditionally, 'gender' has been seen as something that concerns only women. But it has been also due to the lack of large scale data sets which contain questions on work and health for both men and women. Since the mid-1980s we have seen growing calls for the inclusion of men in analysis (see e.g. van Wijk *et al.* 1995). Analyses have begun to emerge, some of the most interesting of which look at changes over time in men's and women's 'roles' and their relative significance for health (see e.g. Hibbard and Pope 1983). However, as indicated earlier, the more specific that gender comparative research seeks to be (within a more quantitative tradition at least), the more it is constrained, not only by theoretical and methodological limitations, but by the fact that at the beginning of the twenty-first century being male or female remains such a key organizational feature of all aspects of our lives, systematically structuring opportunities and experiences. As Emslie and colleagues remarked about their attempt to conduct an explicitly gender comparative piece of research:

attempting to obtain a more homogenous sample of men and women is at best problematic because of the very gendered world we live in; controlling for participation in one social role ... highlights the very different experiences of men and women in other spheres of life.

(Emslie *et al.* 1999: 44)

Sixth, as one part of a move towards greater inclusivity during the 1990s, the call for gender comparative analysis has also led researchers to stress the need to develop measures of work related experience which fully capture the *complexity of the workplace* (Lennon 1987; Matthews *et al.* 1998) *and working life*, with a particular emphasis upon the *quality* and meaning of men's and women's *experience* (see Saltonstall 1993; Simon 1995). For example, van Wijk *et al.* (1995: 600, our emphasis) argue that 'ultimately, the *experienced quality* of each single role and combination of roles seems a far better predictor of health than the sole occupancy of roles' (see also e.g. Dennerstein 1995). It has also been argued that, in order to capture gender related social change, it is important in principle to explore each facet of the paid and domestic work environment (and their combination) for *both* women *and* men (Hunt and Annandale 1993).

Although this mapping of research on the paid work–domestic work combination inevitably over-schematizes what actually have often been contiguous developments, it appropriately depicts the movement of research in the field towards a more inclusive agenda. However, given that it is ultimately the changing social relations of gender which underpin this development, there are in-built limits to how much further research can move forward without reflecting critically upon ways in which gender itself should be conceptualized in research. We turn now to this issue.

Health inequalities and the social relations of gender

In the preceding discussion, we reviewed some dimensions of social change from the perspective of social roles and statuses. However, as raised in the introduction to this chapter, although it is important to appreciate the research advances that have been made from within this framework, it tends to lack an explicit overarching theory of the *social relations of gender* that underpin women's and men's lives. The relatively more fluid movement of men and women between what were once either male or female dominated social spheres is important, but it does not necessarily 'make all things equal' (Hunt and Annandale 1999). The social relations of gender, then, consist of 'more than' movement in and out of social roles; and changes in the occupancy of certain roles and statuses may not mean the diminution of patriarchal privilege, but rather its continuation in new forms. The purpose of this section of the chapter is to step back from the specifics of research findings on gender inequalities in health and to raise a series of broad theoretical concerns. We begin with a brief critical review of the social roles framework.

Next, we consider the gender related social changes outlined earlier from a wider structural perspective that considers changes in the social relations of gender, drawing particularly upon the work of Walby (1990, 1997). We then highlight the issue of *social complexity* through debates between modernist and postmodernist approaches to socio-economic diversity in women's and men's lives at the beginning of the twenty-first century in the west. Finally, we conclude with a summary model of three conceptual approaches to gender inequalities in health as a foundation to a consideration of methodological issues.

Social roles

Criticisms of the use of the social role framework within the sociology of gender are now well rehearsed. In particular, it exaggerates the extent to which social life is scripted or prescribed (see e.g. Connell 1995) and abstracts lived experience from the everyday context in which it is embedded (see Popay and Groves, Chapter 3 in this collection). For instance, there is often an assumption that roles have the same meaning for men and women, whereas, in fact, they may have different meanings for men and women in different social contexts (Clarke 1983). While it is certainly possible to 'correct' for this tendency by building more sophisticated and nuanced measures of women's and men's own interpretations of their circumstances into analyses, they will still be limited if they neglect the wider social relations of gender. Thus looking factor by factor at men's and women's circumstances, as has been the tendency of much research, 'makes it very difficult to pull together a coherent story' to account for relationships between gender and health status (Stein 1997: 117). This ability to develop a 'story' is also exacerbated by the conceptual incoherence that marks the field (Kandrack *et al.* 1994). Thus as Bartley *et al.* (1992) note, we frequently find that variables like marital status, parental status, household structure and occupational social class have been used variously as measures of social role, social position or social conditions. But the most important overall point is that the problems of both factor-by-factor analyses and conceptual confusion result inevitably from theoretical indeterminancy. In brief, it is essential that we move away from treating roles and statuses as properties of individuals and locate them instead in the structural context of men's and women's lives (Arber 1990; Graham 1993; Stein 1997). As Carrigan *et al.* (1987: 167, our emphasis) put it in their critique of the role framework in the study of masculinity (though not referring to health): 'the result of using the sex role framework is an abstract view of the differences between the sexes and their situations, not a concrete one of the *relations between them*'. In the context of our interest in this chapter in gender related social change and health, it means seeing social change as located in power dynamics, rather than as something that 'happens to roles' (Segal 1992; Carpenter, Chapter 2 in this collection).

Changes in the social relations of gender

Dynamic in form, social relations of gender are both responsive to and constitutive of social changes in society that concern men and women. As was stressed earlier in this chapter, the contemporary social relations of gender belie easily summary in terms of 'gains and losses' on the part of either women or men. At the level of subgroups of women and men, new lines of similarity and dissimilarity are emerging, many of which can be conceived of as new axes of inequality. It has been possible to identify several key *areas of social life* within which traditional gender patterns are changing – employment, the family and the household, and education. However, their identification tells us little about the *overall form that patriarchy takes* (as it affects not only women, but also men). Recognizing this, Walby (1990: 174) makes a conceptual distinction between *degrees* and *forms* of patriarchy. Degrees of patriarchy refer to 'the intensity of oppression within a specified dimension' of social life (e.g. the family), while forms of patriarchy refer to 'the overall type of patriarchy' in a society. Taking a broad historical sweep, she argues that British society has shifted in form from 'private' (or domestic) to 'public' patriarchy. This has been associated with the declining significance of domestic activities for women's employment (especially for older women) and the rise in educational opportunities for women. But importantly, while work and education are the spearhead of the shift from a 'domestic/ private' to a 'public' gender order, they are also the leading edge of increased inequalities between women. So while we may be witnessing emerging patterns of equality between some men and some women, this is accompanied by intensified forms of inequality between women (and presumably also between men). This is because segregation is at the heart of public patriarchy, as women are drawn into the public domain but segregated within it. Crucial to this process are the 'spiral of changes' which intersect with age and generation, not simply because they represent 'different stages of the life cycle, but because people of different ages embody different systems of patriarchy' (Walby 1997: 12). This appropriately highlights the fact that relationships between family and household circumstances and health, particularly as they intersect with paid work, are likely to vary considerably for different age cohorts, a topic which has to date been sorely neglected within sociology (see McMullin 1995; Arber and Cooper, Chapter 5 in this collection).

The significance of these points is that, as we build towards more complex models of social change in the lives of men and women in western societies, we need to appreciate that change is unlikely to impact on different subgroups of men and women equally. Age, socio-economic status and ethnicity are among the most important parameters of difference.

Social complexity

The complex and shifting nature of the gender order, as it concerns men as well as women, poses significant problems in the conceptualization of research on health inequalities. Diversity has become the 'buzz word' as we seek to understand newly emerging patterns of inequality which open up new divisions within men and within women, and foster new commonalties of experience between (some) men and (some) women. This new theoretical sensitivity is now central to research on health inequalities, with commentators stressing, for example, the need to embrace the complexity of debate (Lahelma and Rahkonen 1998); to recognize that 'similarity is crosscut by diversity' (Graham 1993: 5); and to appreciate that health varies in response to a 'maze of interlocking variables' (Payne 1991: 115).

However, there is the widely recognized risk that the search for the 'causes' of gender inequalities in health will collapse if the increased recognition of 'sheer complexity' dissipates into relativism. It was only at the end of the 1990s that feminist health researchers began to engage critically with these debates, and to do so quite forcibly. They have been almost wholly neglected within the sociology of men and mascu-linity as it concerns health status. Thus Oakley (1998: 143), for ex-ample, contends that the social world 'remains obdurately structured by a dualistic, power-driven gender system'. This perspective raises very serious concerns about the terms on which gender can be invest-igated when looking at health status. For example, while it seems able to accommodate diversity among women – since a public patriarchy may structure women 'differently' in ways that generate new inequalities – the extent to which we can incorporate a concern with similarities between men and women, and dimensions of male oppression under patriarchy is more questionable. The distinction between sex and gender, as it has recently been open to debate between modernist and postmodern approaches, is central here. Oakley (1998: 135) argues that feminism must continue to use the 'wedge of sex and gender as an oppositional nature/culture dualism to identify an agenda of preventable differences between the sexes, and thus effectively to force open the door of oppres-sion and discrimination'. In similar terms, Doyal (1998), in a discussion of discrimination in women's access to treatment for various health problems, and Scambler (1998) in her discussion of mental health care, highlight the need to retain gender (as well as sex) as a dichotomy in order to recognize the manner in which women are oppressed as 'others' under patriarchy, and the implications that this has for health care. This contrasts to those more sympathetic to postmodern approaches to gender/sex (see Butler 1990; Hood-Williams 1996) who view biological sex as a construction of discourses of gender (i.e. what counts as male and female biological sex is influenced by social and political judgements) and highlight the relative fluidity of gender as it is enacted in everyday life. The postmodern approach to sex/gender is significant insofar as it seems to undermine the structural accounts of gender which are predicated to a significant degree upon dichotomies of sex, gender and (to a lesser extent) masculinity and femininity and the power that attaches to male-sex, male-gender and masculinity. Thus the loss of gender-as-difference in favour of gender-as-diversity becomes problematic for authors such as Oakley, Doyal and Scambler. But nonetheless, they strongly appreciate that the social relations of gender are increasingly complex. Scambler (1998), for instance, echoes many other commentators when she argues that we can understand diversity within patriarchy without rejecting causality and reference to structures. Thus she writes, 'a strong modernism, reinforced by the insights of discourse analysis, offers both an appreciation of difference *and* a structural theory of a patriarchy which is pervasive but chameleon-like in its effects' (Scambler 1998: 107).

In sum, there is here at once a will to be sensitive to the interaction of gender with other factors, that is, to appreciate social complexity while also holding onto gender-as-difference. However, a tension remains in that, the closer we move towards embracing complexity, inevitably the closer we simultaneously move towards undermining the primacy of gender-as-difference (that is, male/female as a binary division of power). Perhaps the solution to this, as Scambler (1998) seems to imply but does not take up in detail, is to conceptualize complexity itself as a product of a new form of gender order – i.e. a causal structure itself – which, rather then being predicated upon the male/female binary, is productive of a more complex and fluid social relations of gender (Annandale and Clark forthcoming). Deploying Walby's (1990, 1997) vocabulary, from such a perspective the new degrees of gender equality and inequality which seem to more radically divide women within specific dimensions of social life, and to draw (some) men and (some) women into circumstances that are more similar than in the recent past in the west, are not the indiscriminate effects of a radical postmodernism, but both the outcome of competing and potentially contradictory forms of patriarchy which concern both men and women. Such an approach would also permit a more inclusive treatment of gender.

As the female-only focus moved progressively to the fore in research on gender inequalities in health during the 1970s and 1980s, men became the new 'shadowy characters' in analyses of the social relations of gender. As Sabo and Gordon (1995: 4) put it: 'while women were in the gender-spotlight, men resided backstage'. However, a cascade of factors has meant that the social production of health and illness among men is now receiving an explicit gender focus which seems likely to culminate in a shift in the methodological approach that is taken to health inequalities. *First, at the theoretical level*, there has been a questioning of patriarchy as privilege within the sociology of masculinity (Connell 1995). This opened the door to the possibility that, far from being health protective, patriarchy may undermine (some) men's health (Annandale 1998b). Thus, in the context of paid work, although patriarchy may operate differently for men and women, its negative health impacts may be the same. For example, Jackson (1994) among others has written of the ways in which work constructs masculinity, undermining health in the process:

> as I piled more and more pressure on myself at work [as a school teacher], my body started to give me warnings that it couldn't stand that alienating rhythm any more. These were mostly in the form of stress-related symptoms like insomnia, an incessant scratching of my scalp when I was anxious, a dry tightening of my throat, tension headaches.
>
> (Jackson 1994: 57)

Second, at the empirical level, the social changes that we outlined in the first part of the chapter, and the new social relations of gender accompanying them, are undermining any straightforward association between women and femininity and men and masculinity. In these terms, many women will recognize Jackson's (1994) description of masculinity, work and its consequences for health as far from male specific. Perhaps the more interesting question, however, is how far many *men* would recognize the equivalent descriptions of the health stresses of domestic and caring work in the home generated by women? Third, arguably the only way in which a gender comparative approach can be addressed is by change at the *methodological level* (see below) which involves including men in analyses alongside women.

To draw together most of the points that have been made so far in the chapter, we conclude this section by outlining in Figure 1.3 three approaches to research on gender and health status, which we have labelled the 'traditional', the 'transitional' and the 'emerging new' frameworks.

These represent broad shifts in the conceptual and empirical research focus over time, from the 1970s to the present day. In Figure 1.3, a hard line has been drawn between the 'traditional' and the 'transitional' frameworks in order to highlight the degree of discontinuity between them. In distinction, the dotted line between the 'transitional' and the 'new' frameworks, highlights the emergence of the 'new' from the 'transitional' framework, that is the continuity between them.

Methodological issues

The bottom (shaded) right-hand box on Figure 1.3 summarizes some of the most important methodological issues which must be addressed if empirical research is to be taken forward within the emerging 'new' research agenda. In the final part of the chapter we take each of these issues up in a little more detail.

As indicated first of all on Figure 1.3, we would argue that a gender comparative approach is essential to the emerging 'new' approach to gender inequalities in health. To argue this point is not in any way to suggest that 'all things are equal', but rather that in times of significant change, it is crucial that we consider the operation of the social relations of gender as they impact on the health of men and women. Although poorly articulated within the 'traditional' framework, it is often automatically assumed that the social relations of gender support 'good health for men' and 'poor health for women'. Thus there is a search for 'what makes women sick' (Annandale and Clark 1996). The emerging 'new' framework moves away from this, to recognize that the social relations of gender operate in much more complex ways. Thus similar circumstances may render *both* men and women vulnerable to ill health or good health. Equally, *similar* social circumstances may produce *different* effects (positive for one, negative for the other) upon the health of men and women – perhaps, for example, because of the interaction of other factors. Thus, it is also important to build an explicit consideration of differences *within* men and *within* women into research. To highlight these points is not to suggest that research on gender and health must always and in every case be comparative, since there may be occasions where it is appropriate to concentrate upon differences within women or men, but simply to highlight the complex ways in which the social relations of gender may impact upon men's and women's health.

This leads us to the second bullet point in the shaded box in Figure 1.3 – the need to explicitly incorporate a concern for the gender order in empirical analysis. In this chapter we have emphasized that this is one of the most pressing concerns in research on gender inequalities in health. Unfortunately, it is also one of the most difficult to take

Figure 1.3 A summary of theoretical and methodological approaches to research in the field

Framework	Theoretical approach	Methodological approach
Traditional	• Only implicit • 'Gender' equals difference between women and men • Distinction between sex/gender • Focus on women's exclusion from/inclusion in social roles and circumstances	• Social roles and statuses as properties of individuals which affect health • Women-only samples • Static • Work and health as predominant focus
Transitional	Growing recognition of • Cross-cutting patterns of gender inequality • Similarities across men and women, and differences within women and within men increasingly emphasized	• Increasingly gender inclusive approach emphasizing diverse axes of inequality • Stress upon the meanings that people attach to roles and statuses
Emerging new	• Explicit attention to the gender order seen as essential • Questioning of the hard division between sex and gender	• Gender comparative • Incorporation of the gender order in analysis • Combination of quantitative and qualitative methods • Emphasis on social change over time in the gender order (in both degree and form) at individual and structural level

forward. The 'traditional' framework, as discussed already, approaches the gender order from the vantage point of roles and statuses, which means that there is little or no sense of gender beyond the level of the isolated individual. In moving beyond this, there are two related ways in which the gender order can be considered more explicitly. The first of these is theoretical; that is, making sure that we have a clear idea of what the gender order consists of and how it may impact upon health in ways that can be specified in empirical research. In qualitative research, which is deductive in nature, this may emerge from data analysis, while in quantitative research which is inductive in form, key concepts and their operationalization will need to be made clear in advance of data collection. Direct incorporation of concepts which tap the nature of the gender order as it may impact upon the health status of women and men has been extremely limited to date. Although in this chapter we have stressed that this is a result of theoretical indeterminancy, the problem is equally methodological and technical. In the words of Herbert Blalock (1964), 'the basic problem faced in all sciences is that of how much to oversimplify reality' (quoted in Stein 1997: 199). Drawing upon the work of Walsh *et al.* (1995), which stresses the need to capture the underlying processes which allocate resources and power in relation to gender, Kawachi *et al.* (1998) have included composite measures of gender inequality at the geographical state level (women's political participation, economic autonomy, employment and earnings, and reproductive rights) in an analysis of mortality and morbidity. They conclude that in the USA, 'women experience higher mortality and morbidity in states where they have lower levels of political participation and economic autonomy. Living in such states has detrimental consequences for the health of men as well' (Kawachi *et al.* 1998: 21). This analysis attends to structure but, as the authors recognize, since their data are aggregate in form (that is, they use age-standardized mortality rates for each state) rather than representing individuals, it risks the ecological fallacy (that is, assuming that the associations that they report would also exist at the individual level). The 'traditional' framework, in contrast, risks the fallacy of composition, that is, assuming that the operation of the whole (the gender order) is equivalent to the sum of its parts (individual roles and statuses). In methodological terms, this brings us back to the theoretical issues that were raised earlier: can we at once take account of social complexity at the individual level while also being sensitive to the form of patriarchy as a social structure?

In Stein's (1997) opinion, progress in this regard has been hindered by the limitations of the dominant positivist method in the field. Referring only to the health of women, but in the global context, she writes that 'positivism can be viewed as a framework that is too constricting to support a broad investigation in women's health and women's lives' (Stein 1997: 209). Health, she contends, has been perceived as having a single, dominant determinant or multiple determinants, when it might be more appropriately approached as 'an intricate, non-linear, tangled web of factors, some of which are socio-political' (1997: 89). Conceptually, Stein's tangled web metaphor is useful since it allows for the social complexity of gender that we have stressed in the chapter. But, as she recognizes, we need to be mindful of its methodological implications:

how do we practically conduct analysis in these terms? Stein stresses that her approach is 'not meant to lead to inactivity, paralysis, or hopelessness', but to move the focus of research from an investigation of 'relatively simple causality to a search for understanding that focuses on synergistic relationships and interactions that may be more fundamental and more reflective of reality' (1997: 172). But, she continues, 'as with many of the critiques of current modes of thought, it is easier to identify the problems and to envision alternatives than to figure out how to operationalise those alternatives' (1997: 208). However difficult these issues are to grapple with, they are an essential foundation upon which the emerging 'new' framework for research on gender inequalities in health must be built, and therefore a central area for methodological development.

Greater use of qualitative methods than has hitherto been the case in research on gender inequalities in health is one important way in which to take account of the social relations of gender alongside the complexity of individual lives. In particular it may permit us to better take account of social agency – how people actively reflect upon their lives and their health and translate this into action (or inaction) (see also Popay and Groves, Chapter 3 in this collection). As Thomas (1999: 11) stresses in reference to the broader area of health inequalities, there has been a tendency to 'shred up' and reduce agency to 'atomised and measurable dimensions of people's knowledge and behaviour' in research – in our terms, in ways that are resonant of the 'traditional' framework. Within the emerging 'new' framework it is important to consider ways in which quantitative and qualitative research can be combined so that we can look in depth at how men and women respond to and actively engage with the gender order in ways that influence their health.

The final methodological component of the 'new' framework is the importance of social change. The 'traditional' framework adopted a rather static or snapshot approach, fixing the lives of women (and sometimes men) in time both conceptually and empirically. But throughout the chapter, we have emphasized that gender structures are changing in ways that are likely to impact differentially upon different subgroups of people, even at the same time as some similarities may be emerging between women and men. It is therefore crucial that we not only try to capture dimensions of structural change in the ways described above, but also change in the life of individuals and subgroups of individuals. A focus upon the individual lifecourse is crucial in this regard (see Arber and Cooper, Chapter 5 in this collection) since it permits us to track the cumulative experiences of different generations (Kuh and Ben-Shlomo 1997; Acheson Report 1998; Bartley et al. 1998) as they vary by gender in the context of other factors, such as socio-economic status and ethnicity.

In conclusion, the purpose of this chapter has been to reflect critically upon the established agenda for research on gender inequalities in health and to outline an increasingly recognized need to establish a new way forward. In particular, we have stressed that social change in various domains of social life, calls for a more gender inclusive approach to research that is sensitive to social complexity, alongside an awareness of new forms of gender related equality and inequality that are emerging both between women and men, and between subgroups of men and subgroups of women. We have concluded by identifying, though not resolving, some of the very challenging methodological implications that follow if this emerging 'new' framework is to lead to greater insights into the aetiology of gender inequalities in health.

Note

1 The term 'economically active' refers to people who are employees, self-employed, participants in government employment and training programmes, and doing unpaid family work. It also includes those aged 16 or over who are looking for work and available to start work within the next two weeks, those who have been seeking a job in the last four weeks, or are waiting to start a job that has already been obtained (ONS 1998: 28). This is self-evidently a wide definition.

References

Acheson Report (1998) *Independent Inquiry into Inequalities in Health Report.* Chairman: Sir Donald Acheson. London: Stationery Office.

Acker, J. (1991) Hierarchies, jobs, bodies: a theory of gendered organisations. in J. Lorber and S. A. Farrell (eds) *The Social Construction of Gender.* London: Sage.

Alvesson, M. and Billing, Y. D. (1997) *Understanding Gender and Organisations.* London: Sage.

Annandale, E. (1998a) Health, illness and the politics of gender, in D. Field and S. Taylor (eds) *Sociological Perspectives on Health, Illness and Health Care.* Oxford: Blackwell Science.

Annandale, E. (1998b) *The Sociology of Health and Medicine.* Cambridge: Polity Press.

Annandale, E. and Clark, J. (1996) What is gender? Feminist theory and the sociology of human reproduction, *Sociology of Health and Illness*, 18(1): 17–44.

Annandale, E. and Clark, J. (forthcoming) Gender, postmodernism and health, in S. Williams, J. Gabe and M. Calnan (eds) *Theorising Medicine, Health and Society: Recent Developments in Medical Sociology.* London: Routledge.

Arber, S. (1990) Opening the 'black box': inequalities in women's health, in P. Abbott and G. Payne (eds) *New Directions in the Sociology of Health*. London: Falmer.

Arber, S. (1997) Comparing inequalities in women's and men's health in Britain in the 1990s, *Social Science and Medicine*, 44(6): 773–88.

Arber, S. and Gilbert, N. (1992) Re-assessing women's working lives: an introductory essay, in S. Arber and N. Gilbert (eds) *Women and Working Lives*. London: Macmillan.

Arber, S., Gilbert, N. and Dale, A. (1985) Paid employment and women's health: a benefit or a source of role strain?, *Sociology of Health and Illness*, 7(3): 375–99.

Bartley, M., Popay, J. and Plewis, I. (1992) Domestic conditions, paid employment and women's experience of ill-health, *Sociology of Health and Illness*, 14(3): 313–43.

Bartley, M., Blane, D. and Davey Smith, G. (1998) Introduction: beyond the Black Report, *Sociology of Health and Illness*, 20(5): 563–77.

Beck, U. and Beck-Gernsheim, E. (1995) *The Normal Chaos of Love*. Cambridge: Polity Press.

Blalock, H. M. (1964) *Causal Inferences in Non-experimental Research*. Chapel Hill, NC: North Carolina Press.

Butler, J. (1990) *Gender Trouble: Feminism and the Subversion of Identity*. London: Routledge.

Carrigan, T., Connell, B. and Lee, J. (1987) Hard and heavy: toward a new sociology of masculinity, in M. Kaufman (ed.) *Beyond Patriarchy*. New York: Oxford University Press.

Clarke, J. (1983) Sexism, feminism and medicalism: a decade review of literature on gender and illness, *Sociology of Health and Illness*, 5(1): 62–82.

Collinson, D. L. and Collinson, M. (1990) Sexuality in the workplace: the domination of men's sexuality, in J. Hearn and D. Morgan (eds) *Men, Masculinities and Social Theory*. London: Unwin Hyman.

Connell, R. (1995) *Masculinities*. Cambridge: Polity Press.

Crompton, R. (1997) *Women and Work in Modern Britain*. Oxford: Oxford University Press.

Crompton, R. and Mann, M. (1994) *Gender and Stratification*. Cambridge: Polity Press.

Dennerstein, L. (1995) Mental health, work and gender, *International Journal of Health Services*, 25: 503–9.

Doyal, L. (1994) Waged work and well-being, in S. Wilkinson and C. Kitzinger (eds) *Women and Health*. London: Taylor and Francis.

Doyal, L. (1995) *What Makes Women Sick?* London: Macmillan.

Doyal, L. (1998) Introduction: women and health services, in L. Doyal (ed.) *Women and Health Services*. Buckingham: Open University Press.

Emslie, C., Hunt, K. and Macintyre, S. (1999) Problematising gender, work and health; the relationship between gender, occupational grade, working conditions and minor morbidity in full-time bank employees, *Social Science and Medicine*, 48(1): 33–48.

Evandrou, M. (1996) Unpaid work, carers and health, in D. Blane, E. Brunner and R. Wilkinson (eds) *Health and Social Organisation*. London: Routledge.

Gershuny, J., Godwin, M. and Jones, S. (1994) The domestic labour revolution: a process of lagged adaptation, in M. Anderson, F. Bechhofer and J. Gershuny (eds) *The Social and Political Economy of the Household*. Oxford: Oxford University Press.

Giddens, A. (1992) *The Transformation of Intimacy*. Cambridge: Polity Press.

Goldthorpe, J. (1983) Women and class analysis, *Sociology*, 17: 483–8.

Graham, H. (1993) *Hardship and Health in Women's Lives*. London: Harvester Wheatsheaf.

Halford, S., Savage, M. and Witz, A. (1997) *Gender, Careers and Organisations*. London: Macmillan.

Hibbard, J. and Pope, C. (1983) Gender roles, illness orientation and the use of medical services, *Social Science and Medicine*, 17(3): 129–37.

Hood-Williams, J. (1996) Goodbye to sex and gender, *Sociological Review*, 44: 1–16.

Hutton, W. (1995) *The State We're In*. London: Jonathan Cape.

Hunt, K. and Annandale, E. (1993) Just the job? Is the relationship between health and domestic and paid work gender-specific?, *Sociology of Health and Illness*, 15(5): 632–64.

Hunt, K. and Annandale, E. (in press) Relocating gender and morbidity: examining men's and women's health in contemporary Western societies. Introduction to special issue on Gender and Health, *Social Science and Medicine*, 48(1): 1–6.

Hunt, K. and Macintyre, S. (1999) Sexe et inégalités sociales en santé, in H. Grandjean (ed.) *Inégalités et disparités sociales en santé*. Paris: La Découverte.

Jackson, D. (1994) *Unmasking Masculinity: A Critical Autobiography*. London: Unwin Hyman.

Kandrack, M., Grant, K. and Segall, A. (1994) Gender differences in health-related behaviour: some unanswered questions, *Social Science and Medicine*, 32(5): 579–90.

Kane, P. (1994) *Women's Health: From Womb to Tomb*. London: Macmillan.

Kawachi, I., Kennedy, B. P., Gupta, V. and Prothrow-Smith, D. (1999) Women's status and the health of women and men: a view from the States, *Social Science and Medicine*, 48(1): 21–32.

Koskinen, S. and Martelin, T. (1994) Why are socioeconomic mortality differences smaller among women than among men?, *Social Science and Medicine*, 38(10): 1385–96.

Kuh, D. and Ben-Shlomo, Y. (eds) (1997) *A Lifecourse Approach to Chronic Disease Epidemiology*. Oxford: Oxford University Press.

Lahelma, E. and Rahkonen, O. (1998) Introduction to special issue, health inequalities in modern societies and beyond, *Social Science and Medicine*, 44(6): 721–2.

Legge, K. (1987) Women in personnel management: uphill climb or downhill slide?, in A. Spencer and D. Podmore (eds) *In a Man's World*. London: Tavistock.

Lennon, M. C. (1987) Sex differences in distress: the impact of gender and work roles, *Journal of Health and Social Behaviour*, 28: 290–305.

Lorber, J. (1997) *Gender and the Social Construction of Illness*. London: Sage.

Macintyre, S. and Hunt, K. (1997) Socioeconomic position, gender and health; how do they interact?, *Journal of Health Psychology*, 2: 315–34.

McMullin, J. (1995) Theorising age and gender relations, in S. Arber and J. Ginn (eds) *Connecting Gender and Ageing: A Sociological Approach*. Buckingham: Open University Press.

Macran, S., Clarke, L. and Joshi, H. (1996) Women's health: dimensions and differentials, *Social Science and Medicine*, 42(9): 1203–16.

Matthews, S., Hertzman, C., Ostry, A. and Power, C. (1998) Gender, work roles and psychosocial work characteristics as determinants of health, *Social Science and Medicine*, 46(11): 1417–24.

Messing, K., Dumais, L. and Romito, P. (1993) Prostitutes and chimney sweeps both have problems: towards full integration of both sexes in the study of occupational health, *Social Science and Medicine*, 36(1): 47–55.

Mills, A. J. and Tancred, P. (1992) *Gendering Organisational Analysis*. Newbury Park, CA: Sage.

Nathanson, C. (1975) Illness and the feminine role: a theoretical review, *Social Science and Medicine*, 9(2): 57–62.

Nathanson, C. (1980) Social roles and health status among women: the significance of employment, *Social Science and Medicine*, 14A: 463–71.

Oakley, A. (1998) Science, gender and women's liberation: an argument against postmodernism, *Women's Studies International Forum*, 21(2): 133–46.

Office for National Statistics (ONS) (1998) *Social Focus on Women and Men*. London: Stationery Office.

Office of Population Censuses and Surveys (OPCS) (1995) *Occupational Health: Decennial Supplement*, ed. F. Drever. London: HMSO.

Pahl, R. (1995) *After Success*. Cambridge: Polity Press.

Payne, S. (1991) *Women, Health and Poverty: An Introduction*. London: Harvester Wheatsheaf.

Phizacklea, A. and Wolkowitz, C. (1995) *Homeworking Women*. London: Sage.

Popay, J. and Jones, G. (1990) Patterns of health and illness amongst lone parents, *Journal of Social Policy*, 19(4): 499–534.

Pringle, R. (1988) *Secretaries Talk: Sexuality, Power and Work*. London: Verso.

Pugh, H. and Moser, K. (1990) Measuring women's mortality differences, in H. Roberts (ed.) *Women's Health Counts*. London: Routledge.

Pugh, H., Power, C. and Goldblatt, P. (1991) Women's lung cancer mortality, socio-economic status and changing smoking patterns, *Social Science and Medicine*, 32(10): 1105–10.

Sabo, D. and Gordon, D. (1995) Rethinking men's health and illness, in D. Sabo and D. Gordon (eds) *Men's Health and Illness: Gender, Power and the Body*. London: Sage.

Saltonstall, R. (1993) Healthy bodies, social bodies: men's and women's concepts and practices of health in everyday life, *Social Science and Medicine*, 36(1): 7–14.

Savage, M. (1992) Women's expertise, men's authority; gendered organisations and the contemporary middle classes, in M. Savage and A. Witz (eds) *Gender and Bureaucracy*. Oxford: Blackwell.

Scambler, A. (1998) Gender, health and the feminist debate on postmodernism, in G. Scambler and P. Higgs (eds) *Modernity, Medicine and Health*. London: Routledge.

Segal, L. (1992) *Slow Motion: Changing Masculinities, Changing Men*. London: Virago.

Simon, R. (1995) Gender, multiple roles, role meaning, and mental illness, *Journal of Health and Social Behaviour*, 36: 182–94.

Sorensen, G. and Verbrugge, L. (1987) Women, work and health, *Annual Review of Public Health*, 8: 235–51.

Stanford, P. (1999) The numbers game, *The Independent Magazine*, 2 January: 13–16.

Stein, J. (1997) *Empowerment and Women's Health: Theory, Methods and Practice*. London: Zed Books.

Thomas, C. (1999) Understanding health inequalities: the place of agency. *Health Variations Newsletter*, 3(January): 10–11.

van Wijk, G., Kolk, C. M. T., van den Bosh, W. J. H. M. and van den Hoogen, H. J. M. (1995) Male and female health problems in general practice: the differential impact of social position and social roles, *Social Science and Medicine*, 40(5): 597–611.

Verbrugge, L. (1983) Multiple roles and physical health of women and men, *Journal of Health and Social Behaviour*, 24: 16–30.

Verbrugge, L. (1989) The twain shall meet: empirical explanations of sex differences in health and mortality. *Journal of Health and Social Behaviour*, 30: 282–304.

Walby, S. (1990) *Theorising Patriarchy*. Oxford: Blackwell.

Walby, S. (1997) *Gender Transformations*. London: Routledge.

Waldron, I. (1991) Effects of labour force participation on sex differences in mortality and morbidity, in M. Frankenhaeuser, U. Lundberg and M. Chesney (eds) *Women, Work and Health: Stresses and Opportunities*. London: Plenum.

Waldron, I., Weiss, C. C. and Hughes, M. E. (1998) Interacting effects of multiple roles on women's health, *Journal of Health and Social Behaviour*, 39: 216–36.

Walsh, D., Sorensen, G. and Leonard, L. (1995) Gender, health, and cigarette smoking, in B. C. Amick III, S. Levine, A. R. Tarlov and D. Chapman Walsh (eds) *Society and Health*. Oxford: Oxford University Press.

Williams, C. L. (1992) The glass escalator: hidden advantages for men in the 'female' professions, *Social Problems*, 39(3): 253–67.

Witz, A. (1990) Patriarchy and professions: the gendered politics of occupational closure, *Sociology*, 24(4): 675–90.

Witz, A. and Savage, M. (1992) The gender of organisations, in M. Savage and A. Witz (eds) *Gender and Bureaucracy*. Oxford: Blackwell.

two

Reinforcing the pillars: rethinking gender, social divisions and health

Mick Carpenter

Introduction: crumbling pillars?

If new life is to be breathed into debates around gender and health inequalities, there is a need for a critical assessment of the theoretical frameworks that underpin research. To this end, this chapter explores the implications of shifts in social and political theory since the rise of second wave feminism in the late 1960s, as part of a wider radical turn in sociology and social policy. This radical turn can be seen as having been built upon 'twin pillars' of analysis, the first of which was a structuralist concept of patriarchy as an institutionalized system of male dominance and oppression of women. Second, it articulated a binary distinction whereby the social inequalities between men and women, including those related to health, were not seen as the product of biologically given 'sex', but socially constructed 'gender' (Oakley 1972). This model can be seen as a powerful and productive framework or 'paradigm' (see Kuhn 1972) within which much research and theorizing about gender and health inequalities have been conducted.

The central starting point of this chapter is that we have now reached the point where the difficulties associated with the 'second wave paradigm' can no longer simply be ignored. This chapter argues that the paradigm should be modified rather than abandoned, while recognizing that there are a formidable range of problems to resolve. First and foremost are a series of difficulties which are not particular to second wave feminism, but to structuralist analysis itself, which Bradley (1996: 1) appropriately dubs 'a crisis in stratification theory'. While gender and class were the central preoccupations of the second wave, from the end of the 1970s other 'structures' of oppression have demanded attention, especially 'race'/ethnicity, disability, sexuality and age. Incorporating these within a structuralist paradigm is at the very least a challenging task, raising the question of whether gender remains a central issue. Alongside this foregrounding of other social divisions has come a challenge to structural analysis itself, particularly from those who, after Foucault, argue that power relations are contingently shaped at the level of daily life through the mobilization of linguistic 'discourses'. Foucault also demonstrated that power over the body or 'biopolitics' is an integral dimension of the social order (see Foucault 1973, 1977; Rabinow 1986). This has been developed by both followers and non-followers into an insistence that society should be seen as 'embodied', undermining the distinction between biology and culture on which the sex–gender duality rested (e.g. Turner 1989; S. Williams and Bendelow 1996). Such an emphasis on contingency and diversity is also associated with claims that capitalist society itself is becoming more fragmented and less fixed, involving a shift to a 'postmodern society' characterized by fragmentation, fluidity and uncertainty. This in turn calls into question the continued relevance of 'grand narratives' such as Marxism and feminism, encouraging eclectic approaches to social theorizing, and particularistic and pragmatic approaches to politics (Lyotard 1984).

In engaging with these issues, my aim is to foster greater theoretical reflexivity in research and argument around gender inequalities in health, by taking a clear position myself and subjecting it as far as possible to tests of evidence. I start by briefly reviewing some of the main issues that arose from the politics of health associated with the New Left and second wave feminism in the 1970s, then outline ways of dealing with them that respond to subsequent postmodern challenges while preserving a viable research paradigm. The final section of the chapter seeks to apply this research paradigm by generating a series of propositions which are both statements about the world and raise questions for further discussion and research.

The feminist second wave and the politics of health

I want to focus first on the influential anthology of feminist and New Left readings brought together by John Ehrenreich in the edited collection, *The Cultural Crisis of Modern Medicine* (1978a), since it encapsulates many of the concerns of this chapter. In particular it shows that socialists and feminists were seeking to grapple with, but also to contain within a

New Left framework, many of the questions which subsequently led to a more concerted postmodern 'cultural turn' in health.

In his introductory essay, Ehrenreich identified and contrasted a conventional 'political economic' or leftist, with an emergent 'cultural' critique of modern medicine, each of which contained divergent viewpoints on the status of medical knowledge and its associated practices. The conventional approach saw medical knowledge as neutral and its practice as actually or potentially beneficial. It challenged (in a North American context) the private ownership of health facilities, and the unequal access to health care of the poor, women and black people. By contrast, the 'cultural' critique broadened the concept of 'the political' by seeing medical knowledge as culturally produced and hence politically contaminated, in two main ways. First, individualist medicine depoliticized the social causes of ill health associated with forms of social exploitation and oppression. Second, medical practice was itself often damaging or iatrogenic, and a means of controlling individual lives by appearing to be scientically based and socially neutral: 'The "scientific" knowledge of doctors is sometimes not knowledge at all, but rather social messages (e.g. about the proper behaviour of women) wrapped up in technical language' (Ehrenreich 1978b: 15). Health care itself was a set of social relationships which also reproduced the class, gender and 'race' hierarchies of the wider society.

Ehrenreich recognized that while the 'political economic' critique emerged from traditional left parties and emphasized a centralized conquest of power and a distributional policy agenda, the cultural critique came from emerging social movements such as feminism, occupational health, black and anti-imperialist movements of the third world. These movements mounted a challenge from below, generating demands for more social empowerment, springing from collective 'self-help' in the present, rather than the traditional left struggle for a future socialist change in management of the 'commanding heights' of centralized capitalism. Such movements also expressed a qualitative critique of contemporary industrial capitalism. For example, the counter-culture of the 1960s challenged the mechanistic basis of western society embedded in its dominant form of medicine and gave greater social currency to eastern holistic views of health and disease processes. Ehrenreich emphasized that intellectual challenges to modern medicine also came from within its own ranks and from an emergent and less subservient sociology of health. Thus, he remarked that Antipsychiatrists such as R. D. Laing (1959) challenged many of the presuppositions of biomedical psychiatry, while in physical medicine stress theorists such as Seyle (1976), Dubos (1959) and others 'stressed a multiple-cause model of disease in which body, mind and environment . . . *interact* to produce disease or to cure it' (Ehrenreich 1978b: 13, original emphasis). The initial departure for radical medical sociology at this time was, ironically, the work of the conservative theorist Talcott Parsons (1950), who argued that medicine *necessarily* controlled the sick and sought to reintegrate them on behalf of society. Within a conflict model of society Parson's approach was 'turned on its head' and linked to the reproduction of exploitative and oppressive structures. However, it was also observed that in contemporary patriarchal welfare capitalism, society became increasingly 'medicalized' as people defined as 'deviant' were encouraged to enter and remain in a dependent 'sick role'. For example, unhappy women were transformed into 'depressives' and gay men into 'sick' homosexuals (Ehrenreich and Ehrenreich 1978).

In recognizing these issues, Ehrenreich was seeking to handle a variety of contradictions. He did not entirely reject political economic concerns about the distribution of medical care, even though cultural analysis often disputed its benefit, because he insisted that it was sometimes beneficial or could be made to be so. Similarly, although he believed that much medicine was culturally contaminated, he argued that an improved social scientific model could be developed which built upon but also transcended the limitations of the mechanistic biomedical model. Though for its time highly sophisticated, in retrospect the diversity of pieces in the Ehrenreich text belied the notion of a unified cultural critique, as opposed to a variety of *critiques* which are not easily synthesized into a common New Left paradigm. From the perspective of the current chapter, however, the most serious deficiency is the unargued assumption that feminist approaches to health can simply be absorbed with the expanded socialist political project. Certainly, by the time of the Ehrenreich anthology in 1978, feminist approaches themselves had become differentiated into 'liberal', 'socialist' and 'radical' strands, with consequential implications for health analysis.

Nevertheless, as Annandale (1998: 63) points out, 'a common feminist vision' around health emerged at this time linking women's health to structures of patriarchal disadvantage. One core element of this was a critical focus on the public–private divide that emerged with modern capitalism, with men dominating the public spheres of market and state, while women's main roles were in the subordinated private sphere of the family. By declaring that 'the personal is political', feminism asserted that what happened between men, women and children in the domestic sphere were also matters of public concern. This in turn implied a challenge to liberal professional ideology that health was primarily a private matter between doctor and patient (even if it was paid for publicly), politicizing both health and the professional encounter itself. In so doing, the feminist emphasis on subjectivity, which disputed the presumed hierarchy between a superior (male) objective reason and an inferior or unreliable and emotional (female) subjectivity, had important implications for the emerging feminist politics of health. Feminism criticized 'scientific' biomedicine for abstracting the body from the person, seeing ill health in terms of a prime pathogenic cause (e.g. a germ or harmful substance like tobacco) disrupting normal bodily functioning. The social implications of scientific medicine were that female patients needed to become passive and 'surrender' control of their bodies to the male physician, so that the physical malfunction could be 'corrected'. The parallel between this and wider patriarchal relations, in which women were objectified and subjected to forms of bodily control, was only too apparent to many feminists. However, the critique had wider implications, leading feminism to become one of the prime protagonists for holistic health approaches asserting the indivisibility of social, emotional and physical influences on health and illness, summed up by the memorable title of the women's self-help 'bible' of the time, *Our Bodies, Our Selves* (Boston Women's Health Book Collective 1973).

The common vision of feminist health analysis and action thus developed a model which showed that medical knowledge represented women in sexist ways, for example in gynaecology textbooks (Scully and Bart 1978). It argued, notably in the 'cultural warping of childbirth', that technological intervention sought to wrest control of traditional areas from women, on dubious therapeutic grounds (Haire 1978). It showed that medicine depoliticized gender relations by defining unhappy women as 'sick'. Ehrenreich and English (1978) showed how historically this was pioneered among the women of the upper classes in the nineteenth century, and others showed how the expansion of contemporary psychiatry drew larger numbers of women into the social control net (Chesler 1972). It was a theory which called on women to struggle together to attack the root causes of patriarchal disadavantage, and to empower themselves in medical encounters, or even to take them over (Ruzek 1980). This critique and struggle against the sick role as part of the wider campaign against professionalism and bureaucracy in modern societies, was not peculiar to feminism, but feminism undoubtedly mounted the most concerted challenges. It is also the case that it has been the most potent, but not always fully acknowledged, force transforming sociology and social policy since the 1970s, not least through the current emphasis on seeing social relations as inherently embodied.

Within this overall paradigm of 'patriarchal disadvantage', however, there have been differences of emphasis between major 'feminisms'. Liberal feminism is associated with the longstanding campaign to achieve formal and substantive equality between men and women in modern, market based societies. It has retained its power in a neo-liberal era, when the heightened emphasis on 'the individual' has facilitated the notion of 'independent women' making incursions into areas previously regarded as male domains. Fiona Williams (1989: 46) argues that it is an approach which does not regard biological differences between men and women as an inherent obstacle to equality, and places particular emphasis on getting women into elite positions in politics, management and the professions as a strategy for change. The focus is more on removing the obstacles to women in the public sphere than challenging the public–private divide as such. Liberal feminism is open to the accusation that its approach primarily benefits a small elite of white, middle class women, rather than the majority. It also tends, according to Annandale (1998: 66), to view the female body and emotionality as 'handicaps' which must be neutralized if women are to emulate male norms.

Both socialist and radical feminism, by contrast, argue that patriarchy is more deeply rooted, necessitating radical change to patriarchal social structures. Socialist feminism disputes Marxism's traditional neglect of gender issues, and its assumption that women's emancipation must await the resolution of the class struggle. As Fiona Williams (1989: 58) points out, this is reflected in efforts to define patriarchy as a semi-autonomous sphere of oppression alongside class exploitation, with patriarchy and class both impacting variably upon the lives of women. Socialist feminism views both men and capitalism as responsible for the exploitation of women's labour in the public and private spheres. It views the welfare state and the health service as at best only partially ameliorative, and at worst, active in reproducing patriarchy (Wilson 1977; Doyal with Pennell 1979).

Radical feminism is diverse, but argues that women are generally exploited as a class by men, for example by processes such as the medicalization of childbirth and women's unhappiness. It tends to foreground biological differences such as male physical strength as explanations of patriarchy, but this varies (e.g. compare Firestone 1971 and Delphy 1984). It thus focuses centrally on the control of women's sexuality and reproductive powers by a patriarchal state and medical profession, and the subjugation of women by male rape, abuse and domestic violence. The main political response advocated by radical feminism is separatist politics, and this is consistent with self-help movements in health which seek to wrest control away from men and assert women's autonomy.

In summary, liberal feminism has put less emphasis than other feminisms on the body and structural power, which underlines its optimism (or what Fiona Williams (1989) critically calls its 'idealism'). Socialist and radical feminism are sensitive to both the physical differences between men and women within accounts of social power based on a sex–gender distinction. Socialist feminists particularly focus on the obstacles that women's childbearing responsibilities have for their entry into the public sphere, and upon the patriarchical ordering of work relations by 'male–female' characteristics (boss–secretary, doctor–nurse). They thus tend to argue for bringing women's private responsibilities into the public sphere, such as through nursery provision, and for the transformation of patriarchal work relations.

Beyond second wave feminism and the New Left

It is possible to acknowledge the combined strengths of the perspectives so far examined, especially socialist and radical feminism, while also acknowledging that they have become problematic. In the first instance, the preoccupation of second wave feminism with the relationship between class and gender has been subject to powerful criticism from black, lesbian and disabled feminists. For example, whereas white feminists campaigned in the 1970s for access to abortion, black feminists argued that this did not acknowledge that black women often had abortions foisted on them (Phillips 1987: 7–8). Some disabled feminists have criticized socialist feminist discourse around community care for opposing the closure of state institutions which many disabled people saw as inherently oppressive (Morris 1991/2). One response to these criticisms is simply to add 'race', disability, sexuality, age, and so on to the number of structures which need to be taken into consideration. As well as being unwieldy, this begs the question as to how this impacts on the lives of individuals, and how divisions are to be 'weighted'. An advantage of postmodern analysis is that it can deal with this by 'decentring the subject', and views people's lives as sites where multiple forms of oppression operate in fragmented and uncertain ways (see Barrett and Phillips 1992). As Annandale (1998: 78) points out, this also reinforces an emphasis on contingency and the notion that patriarchal difference and disadvantage between men and women in relation to health cannot be assumed to be a foregone conclusion.

The chief inspiration for much contemporary poststructuralist analysis is, of course, Foucault. We can acknowledge that Foucault's poststructural analysis of modern medicine, psychiatry and systems of disciplinary power showed systematically how the mobilization of 'expert' discourse of all kinds – medical, psychological and sociological – often involves 'normalizing' power relations over bodies in time and space (Rabinow 1984). Nevertheless, as a general paradigm, not only does it involve an excessively microscopic view of power, but also the critical focus tends to obscure the benefits of the social regulation of health and illness as a means of expanding personal autonomy (Bury 1997: 13). In this context, improvements in life expectancy and historical decline of infectious diseases in advanced capitalist societies (which, as we shall see later, can at least in part be seen as the result of improved knowledge and public health intervention) have had immeasurable effects in widening the scope for human freedom. Contemporary Foucauldians of health have also turned their attention to the social scientific critique of biomedicine and its advocacy of an improved social and holistic causal model. They regard this as a modernist illusion, which they suspect of being linked to a thinly disguised totalitarian project to collectively regulate people's lives in the name of a reified goal of 'health' (e.g. Lupton 1995). This is consistent with a more general postmodern attack on potentially oppressive 'grand narratives'. The point that such critiques of holism have to make is, however, overstated. As we have already seen, New Left and feminist holistic health politics emphasized personal empowerment and autonomy as routes to improved health. Now too often the distinction between ideology and truth is resolved by collapsing them together, and mixed feelings about medicine are dealt with by seeing it as wholly regulatory.

In dealing with these issues, I want to briefly outline a number of possible foundations for a more satisfactory resolution of the issues raised by poststructuralism, which appear to point in broadly consistent directions. These are the social theory of Giddens, the critical realism of Bhaskar and others, the theory of human needs developed by Doyal and Gough, the sociology of emotions and health associated with Freund and others, and the analysis of the gender order associated with Connell. As should become apparent, these offer theoretical paradigms which themselves need to be examined critically, rather than treated simply as templates for the analysis of gender inequalities in health. I would argue however that they are nevertheless sufficiently robust to withstand deconstructive scrutiny.

Two central problems with the postmodern image of society are, first, the articulation of a 'pluralist' view of power as essentially to be negotiated, and second, a fragmented rather than constituted view of human subjects. Giddens' social theory commands attention as one of the most concerted efforts to deal with these issues, combining 'structure and process' in the analysis of social life, and suggesting that society has shifted towards a 'late modern', rather than a radically different postmodern direction. For Giddens 'reflexive modernity' is characteristic of the contemporary period, involving the spread of epistemological and ontological doubt from philosophy into daily life, which makes the contemporary self an uncertain project. This, he argues, represents a continuation rather than a rupture from the critical traditions of the Enlightenment. So does 'a recognition that science and technology are doubled-edged creating new parameters of risk and danger as well as beneficent possibilities for humankind' (Giddens 1991: 28). Implied here is a notion that, though scientific knowledge is socially produced and must be viewed with scepticism, it has a valid core and can potentially be harnessed to social progress. Giddens' concept of 'social structuration' also offers ways of seeing social life as contingent and created from below, while also being institutionally channeled. Moreover, it is underpinned by an ontological view of humans as whole subjects who are both socially shaped and creative agents (Giddens 1984).

I want to endorse Giddens' balanced approach to science which treats its claims to knowledge 'critically', but does not necessarily put it on the same footing as all other claims to 'truth', and also his sceptical but ultimately open perspective on the social applications of modern science. I also wish to endorse his concept of social structuration, and its underlying ontological perspective, while criticizing his particular approach to it as weighted too much towards process and not sufficiently cognizant of structure. Thus critics have argued that, by focusing on agency and the contingent features of social life, and not explaining the tendency of social orders to reproduce themselves, he concedes too much ground to poststructuralism (Layder 1994: 125–9). Additionally, Giddens adopts an idealist approach to 'modernity' which obscures its underlying capitalist momentum. A more appropriate starting point might be Bradley's (1996) insistence that the contemporary world is characterized by contradictory tendencies to both social fragmentation and diversity, and greater social polarization and concentration of power. If social inequalities are in some respects becoming more rigid, as suggested by Westergaard (1995) and others, then this limits the scope for postmodern 'diversity', especially for those who are the losers rather than those who gain within contemporary capitalism.

These issues have been addressed by advocates of a 'realist' or 'critical realist' epistemology, such as Bhaskar (1989), Sayer (1992) and others. They share some of the same concerns as Giddens but in practice arguably achieve a more genuine balance between structure and process, the discursive and the real, and the constraining and the creative dimensions of social life. Realism accepts that the social or natural world must always be approached through theoretical frameworks which do not mirror it as such. Nevertheless, the physical or social world exists independently of theory as demonstrated by the tendency of 'generative structures' to cause events. From the point of view of understanding health and illness, realism allows for synthesis because it makes no fundamental distinctions about the scientific status of medicine and sociology. As with Giddens, there is recognition of the complexity of the social world and a similar commitment to science as an emancipatory project. However, Bhaskar disputes the concept of structuration itself, preferring the notion of 'restructuration', as a corrective to what he sees as Giddens' 'voluntarism', as social contexts often involve pressures on agents to reproduce existing structures (Bhaskar 1983).

This is an admittedly sparse introduction to a complex subject. Its purpose is primarily to outline the approach to be taken in the rest of this chapter. I therefore now want to critically review some theoretical approaches consistent with a realist perspective on gender inequalities in health, starting with the pathbreaking work on health and human needs by Doyal and Gough (1991). This work views humans as inherently active and constituted agents, disputing relativist notions that needs are simply historically constructed. They identify two 'basic needs of persons'; physical health and individual autonomy, with the former as a pre-condition for the latter. Meaningful social participation is also seen as a universal 'basic need'. This means that their theory gives priority to democracy and civil rights as aspects of human needs. After specifying the social and political conditions by which cultures can create the conditions for basic needs satisfaction, they go on to identify what they call the 'intermediate needs' which are universally necessary to ensure that first order basic needs are met and maximized. These include access to nutrition, clean water, physical and economic security, a non-hazardous physical environment, a secure childhood, access to good primary relationships through life, access to appropriate education and health care, and safe contraception and childbearing. They then assess countries across the world according to these criteria, on the basis of which they argue for the reformist welfare state as the best 'satisfier' of these conditions, but with greater decentralization and responsiveness to the wishes of users than in the past. Highlighting their theory as a promising starting point, however, does not necessitate endorsement of all the details, or the precise political conclusions which they draw, as these are a matter of debate (e.g. Soper 1993; Wetherly 1996). One serious problem from the perspective of this chapter is that their universalistic framework fails to focus centrally on gender. For example, the discussion of work hazards identifies only paid work as a matter of concern, and the section on 'childhood security' has no discussion of whether this might mean different as well as similar things for boys and girls.

The recent development of the sociology of emotions is broadly consistent with a universalistic and ontological theory of needs. Just as sociology customarily looked at people in a disembodied way, so the role of emotion in social life was similarly neglected. This has now emerged as a major area of investigation, viewing humans as cognitive and active as well as constrained agents, seeking to connect the somatic or bodily processes within which emotions are embedded, to psychological processes and social relations (Freund 1990; James and Gabe

1996; S. Williams and Bendelow 1996). It can therefore potentially provide the basis for a holistic and realist paradigm from which to approach health and illness, which overcomes artificial splits between body, mind and society. One way it can do this is by utilizing social 'stress' as a mediating concept which has somatic, cognitive (i.e. perceptual or discursive) and social structural dimensions. Thus while early theorists such as Seyle (1976) tended to adopt a mechanistic and deterministic approach (i.e. objective social stressors), cognitive psychology has, in reaction to this, placed too much emphasis on perceptual dimensions (i.e. what is identified as stressful) and thus allows too much scope for agency in relation to stress. Politically, this tends to make stress an individual rather than social responsibility. A structuration model would see stress as inherent in unequal social relations which constrain people's choices, but would not regard people as completely individually or collectively powerless.

The work of Wilkinson (1996), developed theoretically by S. Williams (1998), is promising in this regard, but its failure to consider gender and 'race' inequalities alongside the effects of income inequality is currently a major deficiency. Wilkinson's fundamental argument is that it is the emotional impact of social inequality linked to a sense of injustice, worry and insecurity that has the most corrosive effect on health, operating through mind–body pathways (for example, leading to elevated blood pressure). His other main point is that supportive social relationships (what Doyal and Gough call 'primary relationships') and dense social networks mediate these influences, but that these too are structurally distributed. Looking comparatively, he shows that societies characterized by widening inequality and social fragmentation/individualization (with what he calls declining 'social capital'), most notably the USA, have been slower to reduce general mortality and have poorer records on health inequalities.

Since the theories so far discussed have been generally endorsed but also criticized for failing to give prominence to gender, I will now address how this can be brought more centrally into focus within a realist paradigm. This is what the work of Connell (1987, 1995) promises, though its full potential has yet to be realized. Above all, it offers a means of analysing gender and health that also includes men. Early theorizing on men was often reactive to second wave feminism, suggesting that the 'universal man' was socialized into the sex-role system in ways which, although oppressive to women, also developed men in distorted ways as emotionally repressed and power oriented. This restricted their 'human' self-realization, and was responsible for men's greater risk of early death through suicide, dangerous driving and heart disease (Brannon 1976). Role analysis tends to 'oversocialize' determinism, and a more appropriately structured notion of women's oppression has since emerged. For example, Butler's (1990) 'queer theory' sees 'femininity' not just as an unambiguous social role into which girls are smoothly socialized, but something that must be worked at and acted out with difficulty (involving 'performativity') as it does not come 'naturally'. Connell's work mirrors this shift in feminism by identifying a more variable range of 'masculinities', as ideologies and associated practices linked to other divisions such as class, 'race'/ethnicity and sexuality, with more emphasis on male agency. Thus he identifies 'hegemonic' forms associated with middle and upper class males, 'subordinated' forms associated with the working class, and 'marginalized' masculinities such as those associated with gay men. Connell's model has, however, come under criticism from poststructuralist directions. For example, Hearn (1996) criticizes him for 'reifying' masculinities and failing to draw attention to the enormous individual variety of men's practices and social relations. Nevertheless, Connell's model remains the most robust approach currently available, and offers a useful starting point for analysis of health differences among men.

Having spent some time seeking to reinforce the twin theoretical pillars identified in the introduction to this chapter, it is now time to test out whether they can bear the weight of empirical analysis of gender inequalities in health. My approach will be to continue handling the complexities which, as I have shown, first emerged with the New Left and second wave feminism, rather than lapsing into an atheoretical empiricism or postmodern multicausality. I have argued for a realist framework as the most appropriate means of achieving a balance between structure and process, and analysis of biology and culture, in ways that draws on and seeks to extend the insights of socialist and radical feminism. Methodologically my approach in the rest of the chapter seeks to approximate to what Layder (1998) calls 'adaptive theory'. This is a realist method which seeks to achieve two-way communication between theory and empirical research, by generating 'middle range' propositions which can be connected to broader structures or theoretical systems.

Eight realist propositions on gender and health

There is a need to start from gender, rather than women, and health

Just as feminists were correct to assert that women could not be simply added on to traditional analysis, neither can an analysis of men's health simply be developed alongside women's. As Connell (1987, 1995) argues, in focusing also on masculinity, the gender order as a whole, and men's and women's relation to it, needs to be brought into view. This does not mean that we cannot examine men or women separately, but the *relational dimension* must always be kept in view (see also Chapter 1 in this collection). In this respect, the New Left critique of orthodox Marxism's view of class as an objective category, is still relevant. Most notably, E. P. Thompson, though advocating a materialist approach to history, insisted that 'class' did not exist unless it could be shown to be something which 'happens' in human relationships when workers and capitalists relate together as oppositional communities (Thompson 1968). While Thompson's 'socialist humanist' approach to history rightly put emphasis on active human subjects, he can be criticized for neglecting the ways in which class relations were also shaped from above by capitalists (Anderson 1980), and for failing to foreground gender in his analysis (Kaye and McClelland 1990).

Nevertheless Thompson's general approach is relevant to an examination of gendered social processes and their impact on health. We can see gender as something which must be shown to happen in the way that men, women and children feel and behave towards each other, towards people of the 'opposite' and the same sex. We can predict that this will involve patterned or 'structured' forms of difference which will involve elements of perceived conflict and actual struggles. We cannot, however, predict in advance how these will shape up, nor should we assume that patriarchal relations will be reproduced by men alone. Similarly health and illness must be regarded as key dimensions of the gender order in ways which affect those born male and female throughout their lives, although not in predetermined ways. There are numerous examples that could be given. In traditional and some developing societies girls may be regarded as a burden and neglected or even killed. In more economically developed societies, boys' physical strength may be developed by training and girls' restricted (Connell 1987). Social ideologies and interventions thus impact differentially on males and females.

The biological, social and cultural influences on male and female health are more similar than different

Although social relations of 'difference' and their implications for health and illness need to be a central issue for research, this should not obscure consideration of what is the same for males and females, which might also be the basis for articulating a universalist interest around health. In other words, it is possible to argue for universalism on the basis of evidence that is open to the possibility of difference, while remaining critical of an assumed one that omits any significant reference to gender – criticisms made above of Doyal and Gough (1991) and

Wilkinson (1996). Much of what it is to be human and live in societies is the same for men and women. Our biology is basically similar, with, of course, some important differences. While research into measurable 'sex differences' on children as they mature has been extensive, it has shown a great deal less difference than gender stereotyping imagines, mainly around girls' greater verbal abilities and boys' greater spatial ability (Burr 1998: 27–31). Whether or not the fact that girls may be more articulate, and boys better at catching balls, is a reflection of differences in the brain structures of males and females, they hardly form the basis for the extensive social inequalities that exist between them.

Thus, rather than starting from differences in health, the most striking development is that *both* men's and women's life expectancy in Britain and the rest of the developed capitalist world has improved enormously since the nineteenth century, despite a continuing gap in favour of women (Office for National Statistics 1998: 124). In addition, the kinds of health problems which men and women experience are often similar. Males do have an excess mortality persisting through to later life. They are more at risk of dying in childhood and adulthood from 'accidents and poisoning' and in middle years from circulatory disease (heart attacks and strokes). However, beyond the menopausal years, women's mortality risk from circulatory disease catches up with men's (Office for National Statistics 1998: 135). These patterns are remarkably similar across the western world with some important variations, most notably the much greater excess male mortality in the former state socialist countries of the Soviet Union and eastern Europe (see Chenet, Chapter 7 in this collection).

However, in defending a qualified universalism, there is no scientific excuse for the common practice of regarding men as the standard, and women as different or even deviant. Research which implicitly regards males as the universal gender has customarily been the norm in epidemiological research, and even animal research and drug testing (Carroll 1992: 99). A renowned study in inequalities research, the longitudinal study of Whitehall civil servants in Britain, is often cited as providing general evidence of the damaging effects of hierarchy on health. Yet the first Whitehall Study had 18,000 men and no women. The second study included women, but still twice as many men (Marmot *et al.* 1991). While generalizing from studies based on men is the norm, women's health problems are typically seen as specific to them. Depression is seen as a female problem, a social stereotype to which sociological researchers have unwittingly contributed (Brown and Harris 1978). It has also been suggested that feminist accounts of the psychiatric system as a patriarchal regime of control over women is misleading because significant numbers of men are also regulated by it (Busfield 1996: 230–1). By contrast, heart disease is not typically seen as a 'woman's problem', despite being a major mortality risk, particularly after the menopause (Sharp 1994). Public concerns around cancer among women are mobilized much more towards those specific to them, such as breast and cervical cancer, and much less on other gender neutral forms such as lung cancer, the incidence of which is rising as more women take up smoking, especially in younger age groups (Graham 1996).

There is much 'structured diversity' in health experiences among men and women, as well as between them

I have borrowed the concept of 'structured diversity' from Ginsburg (1992). This takes account of the shift towards analysing fragmentation and social diversity, while at the same time acknowledging the continuing impact of major social divisions of class, 'race'/ethnicity and gender, to which age, sexuality and disability could also be added. In analysing gendered patterns of health, we need to recognize that both men's and women's health experiences may be differentiated in complex ways and that we should not take for granted from the outset that gender will necessarily be the most important factor affecting them.

In a British context, the limited amount of research on gender and health has sometimes looked also at its interaction with social class (or more broadly, socio-economic position), and how this is mediated by domestic position (marital status, children or other caring responsibilities, and so on). This has been broadly consistent with, but not always explicitly stated in terms of, a socialist feminist research agenda. Issues such as 'race' and sexuality have been largely ignored, and are only now beginning to be addressed. Age may have been considered as a 'variable', but not as a relational system of oppression. Research has also often been hampered by the fact that feminist interpretations were being made of data collected within patriarchal paradigms, for example with women's social class often being defined by their husbands' occupation. Arber (1989, 1991) and others have developed an approach which treats men and women as both individuals and members of households, as a better reflection of the complexity of their social identities, and found class gradients in mortality in both instances.

Although this approach adds sophistication, it still tends to use conventional occupational definitions of class which have traditionally informed British research into health inequalities. Attempts to deal with this problem, which include the development of alternative measures such as income, housing tenure, access to cars, and education, are praiseworthy particularly since (see Chapter 1 in this collection) occupational definitions of class exclude increasing numbers of unemployed and so-called 'unoccupied' people such as single parents. These alternative measures also point to the close associations between economic and social disadvantage and poor health (Smith and Harding 1997). However, there remains the question of what structured social relationships underpin them. For example, education may be cited as a feature of structured class disadvantage, or as evidence for the influence of 'lifestyle' and agency. The 'fourfold' heuristic model provided by the 1980 Black Report on health inequalities in Britain (Townsend *et al.* 1992) still often provides the starting point for the realist analysis of inequalities of health. The fourfold model proposed that the differences observed may be: (1) an 'artefact' of the way that statistics are collected; (2) due to processes of biological or social 'selection'; or socially caused by (3) 'cultural behavioural' and/or (4) 'material' influences associated with social position. The Black Report, and much research in its wake, has regarded 'health inequalities' predominantly in terms of questions of class. The question therefore arises as to whether this paradigm can be adapted to the analysis of structured diversity in health. In addition, critics have for some time pointed out that cultural-behavioural and materialist explanations should not be seen as alternatives (e.g. Blane 1985). In other words, The Black Report tends to dichotomize rather than integrate the analysis of structure and agency. Nevertheless, it is useful to investigate the relative extent to which gender health differences over time are products of social selection, changing cultural values and material differences between men and women.

This dichotomy between structure and agency is particularly unhelpful for analysing the influence of 'race' and ethnicity, which are typically absent or marginalized in both 'inequalities' and gender and health research. Traditionally, the sociology of 'race relations' has been divided between radical 'political economic' approaches with strong tendencies to class reductionism of 'black' disadvantage, and approaches which emphasize 'culture'. The latter have tended to be either reformist and 'multicultural', seeing 'culture' in a positive light, or conservative and associated with a 'new racism' (Barker 1981) which explains social and health disadvantage by reference to problematic cultural traits. In the 1990s, the notion of 'black health' which inspired the early studies gave way to a more empirical focus on interactions between biology, culture and political economy. It has become recognized that 'blackness' does not differentiate sufficiently between groups with different origins, such as African Caribbeans, Indians, African Indians, Chinese and Pakistanis/Bangladeshis (Brah 1992; Smaje 1995). While this leaves considerable scope for debate about influences on health, Nazroo's (1997) interpretation of the fourth national UK survey of ethnic minorities, which included a substantial focus on health, still shows strong connections between 'race' and class alongside the influence of ethnic diversity. The results also confirm the interplay of gender and economic disadvantage, most strikingly in the case of Bangladeshi and Pakistani women (Nazroo 1997). Such results vindicate Bradley's (1996) call to analyse both processes of fragmentation and structural disadvantage.

Gendered patterns of mortality and morbidity are not just a statistical artefact

While it is hard to argue that male–female mortality differences are a statistical artefact, it is often suggested that female excess morbidity is, at least in part, socially constructed. One possibility is that 'masculinity' leads men to deny illness out of fear that it displays weakness, and that as a result they are less prepared to report symptoms or use health services than women. It has also been suggested that health professionals and researchers may also be more likely to cast women in the sick role. However, research by Macintyre (1993) into the common cold in fact supports a 'whingeing male' thesis that men report more symptoms, but confirms that investigators expect to find more illness among women. After showing that this finding is consistent with studies of other more serious conditions, she argues that statistics are more likely to underestimate rather than exaggerate women's excess morbidity. This is confirmed by more recent research which suggests that the nature of the condition rather than gender is the main reason for family practitioner consultations (Hunt *et al.* 1999).

However, while research shows that women's excess morbidity is not simply institutionally produced by health services, it does not fully deal with social constructionist issues. A realist perspective would accept that while sickness and disability can be defined only socially, they nonetheless have real social, mental and physical effects. This means approaching it from a number of angles, as in the British General Household Survey, including measures of self-assessed health, and the extent to which people's daily activities (such as climbing a flight of stairs or carrying groceries, see Table 2.1) are limited by health. This relates health to subjective feelings of well-being, and as a means of 'social inclusion' consistent with Doyal and Gough's (1991) theory of need. Blaxter (1991) has shown that these measures are both class and gender related. They have also been related to ethnicity, as shown in Table 2.1. Pakistani and Bangladeshi men and women emerge as one of the most economically and health disadvantaged groups in Britain. Of course the significance of these 'activities' to health should not be taken as read (carrying groceries usually has more significance for women), and much work needs to be done to contextualize the emerging approach to health to people's diverse collective and individual circumstances.

Table 2.1   Selected aspects of health of whites and members of ethnic minority groups

	Self-assessed health fair/poor		Activities limited by health[1]	
	Men %	Women %	Men %	Women %
Whites	26	32	12	22
All ethnic minorities	29	35	12	19
Caribbean	33	39	8	22
All South Asians	29	33	14	18
Indian	26	32	14	15
African Asian	26	27	10	15
Pakistani	34	38	16	24
Bangladeshi	35	41	22	21
Chinese	20	28	12	9

Note: [1] Moderate activities, one flight of stairs, walking half a mile or carrying groceries
Source: Nazroo 1997: 18–23

'Natural' and social selection play a part in gendered patterns of health

One possible explanation for gender differences in health is that women's biology protects against early mortality compared to men, but involves an inherited risk of greater morbidity. While sociological and biological explanations of gender patterns of health have often been in opposition, as Benton (1991) argues, it might be time to cautiously acknowledge the possibility of biological influences on social patterning. Stacey (1988) in particular has also argued for the need to recognize that health has a 'biological base'.

There is some evidence of a female 'natural' advantage in that, while more males are conceived, they are more often spontaneously aborted in humans and other animals (Doyal 1995: 19). There is also a plausible argument that in a period of increasing life expectancy, male sex hormones increase the early vulnerability of men to heart disease, while oestrogen protects women up to the menopause (Waldron 1993). However, there is some evidence contradicting the link between sex hormones and coronary risk (Stacey and Oleson 1993). Yet while sex hormones might affect the uptake of cholesterol, they are a dubious basis for theorizing the behavioural differences between men and women. For example the assumption that testosterone is responsible for male aggression, competitiveness and striving, and other behavioural differences which are associated with a higher risk of mortality from accidents, suicide and violence, and the so-called Type A behaviour that is said to increase male risk of heart disease is, as Rippon (1994: 208–10) suggests, to mistake correlation for cause. The work of Connell (1987, 1995) and others shows that these behaviours are socially produced and reproduced, and they can be shown to be subject to variation across cultures.

Thus the influence of biology is always mediated by social context. For example, in pre-industrial societies any biological advantage that women had was more than cancelled out by the effects of traditional patriarchy. Enforced childbearing, overwork and poorer access to food compared to men meant that women's life expectancy in pre-industrial societies was typically *lower* than men's (Johansson 1977). Capitalist modernity, therefore, in changing the circumstances of patriarchy, also produced a mortality advantage to women in industrialized societies, the reasons for which I now explore in more detail.

Gendered patterns of health and illness are the historical product of 'social structuration'

The previous paragraph made the point that what is taken for granted as a 'fact of nature' is actually a product of history. The implications of this are that gender patterns of mortality and morbidity may not be set in stone and may change again in response to both social pressures from above and agency from below. I want to explore these issues by revisiting the familiar debate between McKeown (1976) and Sretzer (1992) on the reasons why mortality from infectious disease declined with the advance of capitalist modernity in industrialized societies. I argue that while Sretzer's work offers a more satisfactory account on sociological and social policy grounds, neither of them makes any reference to gender, a deficiency which I seek to remedy, focusing solely on the British case.

To briefly recap, McKeown (1976) argues that medical interventions had relatively little impact on mortality. Instead, rising living standards and improved diet conferred greater 'host resistance' or immunity, particularly against the biggest killer, tuberculosis. Sretzer (1992) qualifies this by suggesting that 'exposure' to dangerous pathogens was reduced by state and professional public health interventions and the diffusion of hygienic ideology among the population. Sretzer also makes the important point that rising standards of living were not simply autonomously generated, but were influenced by the agency of social movements such as unions and political parties. Johansson's (1977) analysis (referred to above) enables us to build gender into this debate, as she points out that young women were particularly vulnerable to early death from tuberculosis. However, as well as accounting for the decline in infectious mortality, we need also to explain how gender relates to the rise in differ-ential patterns of mortality and morbidity from modern 'degenerative illness', the other side of what Omran (1971) called the 'epidemiologic transition'. I want to suggest that these patterns were socially 'structurated' by a major shift in the nature of modern industrial life which, drawing on Lewis (1992), I shall call 'single breadwinner capitalism'.

The most dramatic fall in death rates coincided with major social and political-economic change, one of the most far reaching being increased capitalist investment in new mass industries from the end of the nine-teenth century which were increasingly prominent up to the 1970s. The enhanced productivity of such industries appeared to offer the prospect for a male 'family wage' to which many men aspired (but the majority never achieved). This was linked also to 'protective' legislation and norms which confined women to certain forms of work, and increasingly expected them to withdraw from employment to become 'housewives' and mothers. This trend was reinforced by social policy, including the 1942 Beveridge Report and Labour government's welfare legislation of 1945–51 (Wilson 1977). Though male driven, these changes were not simply foisted on women, as there is evidence that the prospect of becoming a housewife appealed to significant numbers of women (Bourke 1994: 64). This dovetailed with other changes, in that rising household incomes reinforced women's desire to have fewer children. Men did not gain as much from this with respect to their physical health. They were still exposed to the physical risks of 'traditional' occupations such as mining and construction. They were also, along with some women, increasingly exposed to the health risks associated with large scale 'mass' work, which resulted from alienating work environments characterized by the 'pressure' to produce and lack of autonomy, lower-ing 'host resistance' to mortality from heart disease and strokes (Marmot *et al.* 1991). There was, however, also a cost for women, in that while the housewife 'role' was associated with cumulative improvements in physical health, the social isolation and denial of self involved in tending to other people's 'needs' increasingly had negative mental health effects (see Brown and Harris 1978; Hochschild 1983).

I am aware that this general argument oversimplifies the diverse social circumstances and responses of real men and women. It also focuses on productive relationships in the public and private spheres and does not examine risks of 'exposure' resulting from harmful forms of consump-tion and 'lifestyle' choices. These too have been patterned by class, gender and 'race'/ethnicity, and it is not necessarily reductionist to suggest that consumption patterns are linked to individual coping mechanisms shaped by structural position. Graham (1987) has shown that women's smoking helps mothers to 'cope' with the mental health pressures of caring for children on a low income, synthesizing 'cultural behavioural' and 'materialist' analysis. Such an approach is in principle extendable to men. Here Connell's analysis is helpful in that it shows the linkages between ideologies and practices of masculinity and class relations. Type A behaviour, for example, is most often associated with the 'hegemonic' masculinity of higher class males, who in fact now have a lower risk of coronary disease (Johnston *et al.* 1987). 'Subordinated' forms of masculinity, and the coping behaviours associated with them including greater risk taking, are linked to structural position, and may reinforce the higher mortality associated with it (Waldron 1993).

It is possible to acknowledge that changes have occurred in social patterns of production and consumption since the 1970s without proposing that capitalist societies have dissolved into postmodernity. Feminism continues to challenge male breadwinner prerogatives at a time when contemporary capitalism is less able or willing to provide access to secure and well paid work. At the same time, work itself has shifted more to services in Europe and North America, which makes 'emotional labour' (dealing with the needs of others, while suppressing one's own) a significant source of stress within the public sphere (Hochschild 1983). More women are entering paid work, usually in part-time and/or lower paid jobs, and older men, and younger men with few qualifications, are being displaced (see also Chapters 1 and 4 in this collection). These are major changes which may have complex gender, 'race' and class effects on health. The work of Martin (1993) on the increasing tendency to individualize issues around risk and immunity is promising in this respect and corresponds to Giddens' (1991) emphasis on the self as an increasingly reflexive and uncertain project. It could be that women's more active 'coping styles' (Health Education Authority 1995) are generally more adaptive to new capitalist conditions of 'flexible accumulation' than many men's, yet this also depends crucially on the resources available to women of different classes (Arber 1989, 1991). However, a structuralist perspective on these changes is necessary if we are not to imagine that all the problems of late capitalist modernity can be dealt with by better stress management techniques, New Age philosophy, exercise and healthy eating.

Social relations can have positive or negative health effects

The possibility that social relations may have either a positive or negative effect on health follows from the earlier emphasis on the sociology of emotions and social network theory. Unfortunately the available evidence is still often only suggestive and prone to crude ecological fallacies, such as that 'marriage protects' health. Nevertheless, on the positive side, the available evidence does support the Doyal and Gough (1991) thesis that humans need autonomy, close personal relationships and opportunities for social participation. The Alameda County study in the USA (Berkman and Syme 1979) was the first major study to demonstrate this, although the evidence needs placing in a reflexive framework. While social network theory is a powerful critique of a methodologically individualist view of immunity and health associated with the New Right, consistent with the new political emphasis on 'social inclusion', Levitas (1996) has shown that this discourse often expresses a Durkheimian integrationism, which is more concerned to integrate people into modified structures of inequality, than to recognize the need for transformation.

We can radicalize such discourses if, without being overly romantic, we see 'community' not just as a stabilizing force, but as oppositional agency mobilized from below in relation to the market and dominant groups. Historically, subordinated groups developed social networks to oppose or mitigate the effects of industrial capitalism (Thompson 1968). At around the turn of the twentieth century, for example, Jewish mothers in East London played a significant part in combating the effects of poverty on the health of their children (Marks 1990). In the contemporary era in industrialized countries, the social networks of gay men have sought to combat the homophobia accompanying AIDS and have helped to stem its spread. The women's movement has also sought to develop communal networks of practical and emotional support, challenging patriarchy on a variety of fronts and levels, examples of which include women's refuges and rape crisis centres.

However, before waxing too lyrical, we need also to recognize that oppressive and exploitative social relationships can also have damaging effects on health and that sometimes, as a character in Sartre's play *In Camera* put it, 'hell is other people'. Thus in a chapter of this kind, it is important to draw attention to the fact that oppression, violence and abuse by men, as foregrounded by radical feminism, is a community health risk. For example, male sexual abuse of children is emerging as a significant policy issue, and it is consistent with Connell's (1987, 1995) emphasis on patriarchy as associated with hierarchies among men to see them too as victims of bullying, harassment and violence, which may be further compounded by racism and homophobia (Stanko 1994; Pringle 1995). While research has often seen men as sources of 'social support' (e.g. Brown and Harris 1978), more recent research by Oakley and Rigby (1998) has shown that some women perceive that living with men can have negative effects on their own and their children's health.

Women's advantage in life expectancy is a mixed blessing?

> A shorter life expectancy: there's one great inequality men can brandish on their placards, can grumble about to women, who endure most of the others. But perhaps even in this women – as the ones left painfully behind while their husbands move beyond pain – end up suffering the most.
>
> (Morrison 1993: 167)

I am deliberately finishing, briefly, with a proposition which is also a question. As Morrison suggests, men's early mortality is sometimes depicted as evidence that men are increasingly the disadvantaged gender. Increased life expectancy does have some implications for both second wave and postmodern feminism, in that whatever the problems women have experienced with modernity, it has been associated with substantial gains on the past.

Yet on closer examination, the advantage may not be as great as it appears, if quality as well as quantity of life is taken into account. In fact, the risk of greater 'morbidity' which women experience is a lifetime issue, though its nature does change. Thus Macintyre *et al.* (1996) review evidence which shows that women reported more 'malaise' or psychosocial symptoms at all ages than men, but that in older age physical disability becomes more significant for women. Even so we must be careful of overgeneralizing as, despite Morrison's assertion, widowhood can be associated with 'a new lease of life'. Age itself is also a social relation which has been characterized by 'structured dependency' in that ageism interacts with lifetime social disadvantage (Macnicol 1990). Arber and Cooper (1999) have also shown how this is strongly related to social class position. Consistent with the approach taken by this chapter, however, is that the focus on gender and class also needs broadening to embrace other issues such as 'race' and ethnicity.

Concluding comments: strengthened pillars?

This chapter has tried to show the benefits of a theoretically informed and empirically grounded approach to gender inequalities of health, which places contemporary developments in a historical and sociological context. It has suggested that a 'critical realist' approach can enable us to adapt rather than to abandon the twin pillars, in order to develop a more sensitive structuralist analysis of health inequality, and a more sophisticated investigation of the complex interactions between biology and culture. Although much has changed since the late 1960s, I have argued that structuralist perspectives on society, and holistic and humanistic conceptions of health needs, remain indispensable instruments of the research toolkit for gaining a better understanding, and for developing improved social interventions, around gender inequalities of health. I have also suggested that while postmodern challenges can help us to sharpen our existing tools, and may even add new conceptual items of equipment, if seen as alternatives to 'modernist' analysis, they can fall into a number of 'traps'. These include presenting an exaggerated picture of the extent to which contemporary society has moved in socially diverse and more fluid directions; fostering the anthropomorphic fallacy associated with extreme forms of social constructionism which posit that body and nature have no independent existence beyond discourse; and, by failing to give due credit to the gains associated with modernity, encouraging an undue pessimism about the possibility of making significant progress towards a more equal and just social order. I have tried to be alert to the problems associated with second wave feminism, but have also sought to show that it was often more sophisticated than it is sometimes given credit for. Above all, I have sought, within the space available in a relatively short chapter, to test the modified paradigm against the evidence offered by the empirical world.

Acknowledgements

I am grateful to the editors and to Steve Anelay for helpful comments on earlier drafts of this chapter.

References

Anderson, P. (1980) *Arguments within English Marxism*. London: Verso.

Annandale, E. (1998) *The Sociology of Health and Medicine: A Critical Introduction*. Cambridge: Polity Press.

Arber, S. (1989) Gender and class inequalities in health: understanding the differentials, in J. Fox (ed.) *Health Inequalities in European Countries*. Aldershot: Gower.

Arber, S. (1991) Class, paid employment and family roles: making sense of structural disadvantage, gender and health status, *Social Science and Medicine*, 32(4): 425–36.

Arber, S. and Cooper, H. (1999) Gender differences in later life: the new paradox?, *Social Science and Medicine*, 48(1): 1–16.

Barker, M. (1981) *The New Racism*. London: Junction Books.

Barrett, M. and Phillips, A. (eds) (1992) *Destabilizing Theory*. Cambridge: Polity Press.

Benton, T. (1991) Biology and social science: why the return of the repressed should be given a (cautious) welcome, *Sociology*, 25(1): 1–29.

Berkman, S. L. and Syme, S. L. (1979) Social networks, host resistance and mortality: a nine year follow up study of Alameda County residents, *American Journal of Epidemiology*, 109: 186–204.

Bhaskar, R. (1983) Beef, structure and place: notes from a critical naturalist perspective, *Journal for the Theory of Social Behaviour*, 13: 81–95.

Bhaskar, R. (1989) *Reclaiming Reality: A Critical Introduction to Contemporary Philosophy*. London: Verso.

Blane, D. (1985) An assessment of the Black Report's explanation of health inequalities, *Sociology of Health and Illness*, 7(3): 423–45.

Blaxter, M. (1991) *Health and Lifestyles*. London: Routledge.

Boston Women's Health Book Collective (1973) *Our Bodies, Our Selves*. New York: Simon and Schuster.

Bourke, J. (1994) *Working Class Cultures in Britain*. London: Routledge.

Bradley, H. (1996) *Fractured Identities: Changing Patterns of Inequality*. Cambridge: Polity Press.

Brah, A. (1992) Difference, diversity and differentiation, in J. Donald and A. Rattansi (eds) *'Race', Culture and Difference*. London: Sage.

Brannon, R. (1976) The male sex-role: our culture's blueprint of manhood and what it's done for us lately, in D. David and R. Brannon (eds) *The Forty-Nine Per Cent Majority*. Reading, MA: Addison-Wesley.

Brown, G. W. and Harris, T. (1978) *Social Origins of Depression: A Study of Psychiatric Disorder in Women*. London: Tavistock.

Burr, V. (1998) *Gender and Social Psychology*. London: Routledge.

Bury, M. (1997) *Health and Illness in a Changing Society*. London: Routledge.

Busfield, J. (1996) *Men, Women and Madness: Understanding Gender and Mental Disorder*. London: Macmillan.

Butler, J. (1990) *Gender Trouble: Feminism and the Subversion of Identity*. London: Routledge.

Carroll, D. (1992) *Health Psychology: Stress, Behaviour and Disease*. London: Falmer.

Chesler, P. (1972) *Women and Madness*. New York: Doubleday.

Connell, R. W. (1987) *Gender and Power*. Cambridge: Polity Press.

Connell, R. W. (1995) *Masculinities*. Cambridge: Polity Press.

Delphy, C. (1984) *Close to Home: A Materialist Analysis of Women's Oppression*. London: Hutchinson.

Doyal, L. (1995) *What Makes Women Sick: Gender and the Political Economy of Health*. London: Macmillan.

Doyal, L. and Gough, I. (1991) *A Theory of Human Need*. London: Macmillan.

Doyal, L. with Pennell, I. (1979) *The Political Economy of Health*. London: Pluto.

Dubos, R. (1959) *The Mirage of Health: Utopian Progress and Biological Change*. New York: Anchor.

Ehrenreich, B. and English, D. (1978) The 'sick' women of the upper classes, in J. Ehrenreich (ed.) *The Cultural Crisis of Modern Medicine*. New York: Monthly Review Press.

Ehrenreich, J. (ed.) (1978a) *The Cultural Crisis of Modern Medicine*. New York: Monthly Review Press.

Ehrenreich, J. (1978b) Introduction: the cultural crisis of modern medicine, in J. Ehrenreich (ed.) *The Cultural Crisis of Modern Medicine*. New York: Monthly Review Press.

Ehrenreich, J. and Ehrenreich, B. (1978) Medicine and social control, in J. Ehrenreich (ed.) *The Cultural Crisis of Modern Medicine*. New York: Monthly Review Press.

Firestone, S. (1971) *The Dialectic of Sex*. London: Jonathan Cape.

Foucault, M. (1973) *The Birth of the Clinic: An Archaeology of Medical Perception*. London: Tavistock.

Foucault, M. (1977) *Discipline and Punish: The Birth of the Prison*. New York: Vintage.

Freund, P. (1990) The expressive body: a common ground for the sociology of emotions and health and illness, *Sociology of Health and Illness*, 12(4): 454–77.

Giddens, A. (1984) *The Constitution of Society*. Cambridge: Polity Press.

Giddens, A. (1991) *Modernity and Self-Identity: Self and Society in the Late Modern Age*. Cambridge: Polity Press.

Ginsburg, N. (1992) *Divisions of Welfare*. London: Sage.

Graham, H. (1987) Women's smoking and family health, *Social Science and Medicine*, 25(1): 47–56.

Graham, H. (1996) Smoking prevalence among women in the European Community 1950–1990, *Social Science and Medicine*, 43(2): 243–54.

Haire, D. (1978) The cultural warping of childbirth, in J. Ehrenreich (ed.) *The Cultural Crisis of Modern Medicine*. New York: Monthly Review Press.

Health Education Authority (HEA) (1995) *A Survey of the UK Population: Part 1*. London: HEA.

Hearn, J. (1996) Is masculinity dead? A critique of the concept of masculinity/masculinities, in M. Mac an Ghaill (ed.) *Understanding Masculinities: Social Relations and Cultural Arenas*. Buckingham: Open University Press.

Hochschild, A. (1983) *The Managed Heart: Commercialization of Human Feeling*. Berkeley, CA: University of California Press.

Hunt, K., Ford, G., Harkins, L. and Wyke, S. (1999) Are women more ready to consult than men? Gender differences in family practitioner consultation for common chronic conditions', *Journal of Health Services Research and Policy*, 4(2): 96–100.

James, V. and Gabe, J. (1996) Connecting emotions and health, in V. James and J. Gabe (eds) *Health and the Sociology of Emotions*. Oxford: Blackwell.

Johansson, S. R. (1977) Sex and death in Victorian England: an examination of age- and sex-specific death rates, in M. Vicinus (ed.) *A Widening Sphere: Changing Roles of Victorian Women*. London: Methuen.

Johnston, D. W., Cook, D. G. and Shaper, A. G. (1987) Type A behaviour and ischaemic heart disease in middle aged British men, *British Medical Journal*, 295: 86–9.

Kaye, H. and McClelland, K. (eds) (1990) *E. P. Thompson: Critical Perspectives*. Cambridge: Polity Press.

Kuhn, T. (1972) *The Structure of Scientific Revolutions*, 2nd edn. Chicago: University of Chicago Press.

Laing, R. D. (1959) *The Divided Self*. London: Tavistock.

Layder, D. (1994) *Understanding Social Theory*. London: Sage.

Layder, D. (1998) *Sociological Practice: Linking Theory and Social Research*. London: Sage.

Levitas, R. (1996) The concept of social exclusion and the new Durkheimiam hegemony, *Critical Social Policy*, 16: 5–20.

Lewis, J. (1992) Gender and the development of welfare regimes, *Journal of European Social Policy*, 2(2): 159–74.

Lupton, D. (1995) *The Imperative of Health: Public Health and the Regulated Body*. London: Sage.

Lyotard, J. (1984) *The Postmodern Condition: A Report on Knowledge*. Manchester: Manchester University Press.

Macintyre, S. (1993) Gender differences in the perceptions of common cold symptoms, *Social Science and Medicine*, 36(1): 14–20.

Macintyre, S., Hunt, K. and Sweeting, H. (1996) Gender differences in health: are things really as simple as they seem?, *Social Science and Medicine*, 42(2): 617–24.

McKeown, T. (1976) *The Role of Medicine: Dream, Mirage or Nemesis?* London: Nuffield Provincial Hospitals Trust.

Macnicol, J. (1990) Old age and structured dependency, in M. Bury and J. Macnicol (eds) *Aspects of Ageing: Essays on Social Policy and Old Age*. Egham, Surrey: Royal Holloway and Bedford New College.

Marks, L. (1990) 'Dear Old Mother Levy's': the Jewish Maternity Home and Sick Rooms Help Society 1895–1939, *Social History of Medicine*, 3: 61–87.

Marmot, M. G., Davey Smith, G., Stansfield, S. *et al.* (1991) Health inequalities among British civil servants: the Whitehall II Study, *Lancet*, 337:1387–93.

Martin, E. (1993) Histories of immune systems, *Culture, Medicine and Society*, 17(1): 67–76.

Morris, J. (1991/2) 'Us and them'? Feminist research, community care and disability, *Critical Social Policy*, 11(3): 22–39.

Morrison, B. (1993) *And When Did You Last See Your Father?* London: Granta.

Nazroo, J. Y. (1997) *The Health of Britain's Ethnic Minorities*. London: Policy Studies Institute.

Oakley, A. (1972) *Sex, Gender and Society*. London: Temple Smith.

Oakley, A. and Rigby, A. S. (1998) Are men good for the welfare of women and children?, in J. Popay, J. Hearn and J. Edwards (eds) *Men, Gender Divisions and Welfare*. London: Routledge.

Office for National Statistics (ONS) (1998) *Social Trends 28*. London: Stationery Office.

Omran, A. R. (1971) The epidemiologic transition: a theory of the epidemiology of population change. *Millbank Memorial Fund Quarterly*, 49: 309–38.

Parsons, T. (1950) *The Social System*. New York: Free Press.

Phillips, A. (1987) *Divided Loyalties: Dilemmas of Sex and Class*. London: Virago.

Pringle, K. (1995) *Men, Masculinities and Social Welfare*. London: UCL Press.

Rabinow, P. (1986) *The Foucault Reader*. Harmondsworth: Penguin.

Rippon, G. (1994) Sex and gender differences: issues for psychopathology, in D. Tantam and M. Birchwood (eds) *Seminars in Psychology and the Social Sciences*. London: Gaskell.

Ruzek, S. (1980) *The Women's Health Movement: Feminist Alternatives to Medical Control*. London: Praeger.

Sayer, A. (1992) *Method in Social Science: A Realist Approach*, 2nd edn. London: Routledge.

Scully, D. and Bart, P. (1978) A funny thing happened on the way to the orifice: women in gynaecology textbooks, in J. Ehrenreich (ed.) *The Cultural Crisis of Modern Medicine*. New York: Monthly Review Press.

Seyle, H. (1976) *The Stress of Life*, 2nd edn. New York: McGraw-Hill.

Sharp, I. (ed.) (1994) *Coronary Heart Disease: Are Women Special?* London: National Forum for Coronary Heart Disease Prevention.

Smaje, C. (1995) *Health, 'Race' and Ethnicity*. London: Kings Fund.

Smith, J. and Harding, S. (1997) Mortality of women and men using alternative classifications, in F. Drever and M. Whitehead (eds) *Health Inequalities: Decennial Supplement*. London: Stationery Office.

Soper, K. (1993) A theory of human need, *New Left Review*, 197(Jan–Feb): 113–28.

Sretzer, S. (1992) Mortality and the public health 1815–1914, *ReFresh*, spring: 1–4.

Stacey, M. (1988) *The Sociology of Health and Healing*. London: Unwin Hyman.

Stacey, M. and Olesen, V. (1993) Introduction, *Social Science and Medicine*, 36(1): 1–5.

Stanko, E. A. (1994) Challenging the problem of men's individual violence, in T. Newburn and E. A. Stanko (eds) *Just Boys Doing Business: Men, Masculinities and Crime*. London: Routledge.

Thompson, E. P. (1968) *The Making of the English Working Class*. Harmondsworth: Penguin.

Townsend, P., Davidson, N. and Whitehead, M. (1992) *Inequalities in Health: The Black Report – The Health Divide*. Harmondsworth: Penguin.

Turner, B. S. (1989) *The Body and Society: Explorations in Social Theory*, 2nd edn. Oxford: Blackwell.

Waldron, I. (1993) Recent trends in sex mortality ratios for adults in developed countries, *Social Science and Medicine*, 36(4): 451–62.

Westergaard, J. (1995) *Who Gets What? The Hardening of Class Inequality in the Late Twentieth Century*. Cambridge: Polity Press.

Wetherly, P. (1996) Basic needs and social policies, *Critical Social Policy*, 46(16): 45–65.

Wilkinson, R. G. (1996) *Unhealthy Societies: The Afflictions of Inequality*. London: Routledge.

Williams, F. (1989) *Social Policy: A Critical Introduction*. Cambridge: Polity Press.

Williams, S. (1998) 'Capitalizing' on emotions? Rethinking the inequalities in health debate, *Sociology*, 32(1): 121–39.

Williams, S. and Bendelow, G. (1996) Emotions, health and illness: the 'missing link' in medical sociology?, in V. James and J. Gabe (eds) *Health and the Sociology of Emotions*. Oxford: Blackwell.

Wilson, E. (1977) *Women and the Welfare State*. London: Tavistock.

three

'Narrative' in research on gender inequalities in health

Jennie Popay and Keleigh Groves

Introduction

This chapter is concerned to explore the potential for life narratives – the personal 'stories' of individual women's and men's experiences – to shift the contours of inquiry in research on gendered patterns of health and illness. Other contributors to this volume are seeking to problematize the main storyline – 'the men die, women get sick' narrative – as part of a rapidly developing critique of past research in this field. One of the prominent elements of this critique is a questioning of the notion that the patterns of mortality and morbidity among women and men reported in much research in industrialized nations are appropriately described as gender inequalities. There is a growing concern to foreground differences among men and women rather than divisions between them. In the context of recent political and theoretical developments, researchers are seeking to acknowledge and better understand the capacity that individual women and men have to act creatively on and in their lives – their agency. Qualitative research methods are increasingly being used to explore these axes of difference in this and other fields. However, in this chapter we argue that qualitative research, focusing on the accounts that people give of their daily lives and health experiences, offers a means of exploring the relationship between agency and structures – that is between difference and divisions. In so doing, we suggest, this type of research points to the way in which patriarchal ideologies and structures – albeit alongside and interacting with other social divisions – continue to mould women's and men's lives differently. In consequence, we suggest, these processes generate gendered inequalities in health – in the sense that these patterns are socially produced and avoidable.

In developing our arguments we have drawn on a body of qualitative research which is limited in two important ways. First, much of it includes only women in its frame; there is very little research concerned to explore men's subjective accounts of their lives and the experience of health and illness. Second, that which does include both women and men most often does so from a perspective which has been termed difference focused rather than division led. In other words gender (and class) is present in research as a differentiating variable, rather than as a social category embedded in unequal social relationships (F. Williams 1999). In exploring the ways in which qualitative research might recast our knowledge of gender inequalities, we have therefore had to draw on a small number of studies and can only point tentatively to the insights that this research might have to offer.

We begin our chapter by reviewing briefly the 'story so far' in relation to gender inequalities in health in terms of both theoretical and methodological orientations. This allows us to place our emphasis on the role of narrative based research in the context of the wider tradition of scholarship in this field. We then develop our argument for the role of qualitative research which generates narrative accounts of individual experience. Finally, we look in more detail at the potential contribution such research has to make to our understanding of the gendered experience of health and illness.

The story so far?

The emergence of a gender focus in health research

The dominant understanding of gender inequalities in health has been of higher premature mortality rates for most causes of death for men under 50 compared to women in these age groups, and higher rates of non-life-threatening illness (often termed 'minor') for women compared to men at most ages. However, the development of this 'men die, women get sick' storyline about gender inequalities in health is relatively recent and can be traced back to the 1970s. Previously, empirical research into the social patterning of health had focused overwhelmingly on mortality (rather than morbidity) patterns among groups of people living in different socio-economic circumstances.

This longer tradition of social inquiry into population mortality patterns began initially in the nineteenth century and was concerned with spatial variations (even down to differences between different streets) and patterns among crudely differentiated occupational groups. As the Registrar General's classification of occupational social class was developed, this became the dominant mode of categorizing people in the UK, with somewhat different traditions evolving in other countries, notably a focus on educational attainment in the USA (Arber 1990). It is also important to note that, despite the contemporary concern that men's health has been relatively neglected, much research into health experience in general, and social class inequalities in health in particular, has primarily focused on patterns among men, and remains to some extent so focused today (Rosser 1994). Detailed analysis of mortality rates among women in different social classes has often been excluded, usually on the ground that the allocation of social class to women is problematic and many large clinical trials have been based on all male samples.

However, in the 1970s, coinciding with second wave feminism, there was a rapid expansion in scholarship aiming to explore and understand male–female differences in health and illness. This inspired a massive collection and/or analysis of quantitative data from large scale surveys, particularly in the USA and was concerned primarily with morbidity experience. This work consistently reported a morbidity excess among women compared to men – a pattern which contrasted starkly with the mortality excess among men evident in most richer nations. This general pattern has now been reported for North America, many European countries, Australia and New Zealand. It was most powerfully portrayed in Verbrugge's memorable comment when she described patterns of ill health as an iceberg (Verbrugge 1977a, 1977b). She argued that the top and most visible part of this iceberg was made up of mortality and it had a strongly masculine hue, but that the less visible bulk of the iceberg of non-life-threatening physical and psychological illness had a strongly female hue. In most countries where they have been reported, these gendered patterns of mortality and morbidity at a population level are linked to differences in the life expectancy of men and women. In the UK, for example, the average man in England and Wales can expect to live to age 73 – five and a half years less than the average woman.

As the contributions in this book demonstrate, this pervasive grand narrative in gender inequalities research is currently being recast. This is in part a response to changes in life expectancy and in population patterns of mortality and morbidity for major diseases. It is also a response to a growing critique of the dominant methodological and theoretical frameworks informing research on gender inequalities.

Time trends in mortality and morbidity

Annandale (1998) has reviewed the data on the changing epidemiological patterns of mortality among women and men in the UK. On the basis of this analysis, she argues that, although tentative and speculative, the evidence points towards a closing mortality gap between women and men and therefore, by implication, in morbidity from serious life-threatening diseases. This, she suggests, appears to be due to a reduction in male mortality rates rather than a worsening in mortality among women – although in some instances, such as lung cancer and coronary heart disease, there is evidence of a worsening trend among women.

It is not possible to map changes over time in relation to gender differences in 'minor' morbidity and disability in the same way as it is with mortality data. This is partly because of the many different ways in which 'minor' morbidity and disability are measured in research and, perhaps most crucially, because many of the data are based on self-reports. It is therefore not capturing an objectively measurable single state of health and illness – like death – but rather a diverse landscape of subjectively perceived experiences. This has led to the widespread conclusion that, over and above any differences in underlying morbidity, the findings of research reflect differential reporting behaviour among women and men, although in a detailed analysis of the responses of women and men to different types of questions about chronic health problems, Macintyre and colleagues (1999) conclude that there is no evidence that women are simply more likely than men to report ill health. In fact, a great deal of research has reported multifaceted patterns of self-reported morbidity and disability among women and men rather than focusing on a single overarching trend (see e.g. Popay *et al.* 1993; Macintyre *et al.* 1999). It has to be said, however, that these findings have had relatively little impact on the dominant belief that women are sicker than men (Macintyre *et al.* 1996). At the risk of compounding these problems, the evidence does suggest to us that over time women have appeared to be consistently more likely to report higher rates of psychological distress than men (however it is measured) and, while women may not be 'sicker' than men in any general sense, there are consistently large and statistically significant female excesses in relation to single 'symptoms' such as tiredness, headaches, musculoskeletal problems and chronic pain. As we argue below, patterns such as these may offer important theoretical purchase on our understanding of the relationship between gender inequalities and health experience.

The emerging critique of gender inequalities research

Alongside the recognition that, at least in terms of mortality, patterns among women and men are changing over time, the dominant methodological and theoretical frameworks informing much past research on gender inequalities in health have been the subject of increasing criticism. There are at least three dimensions to these critiques: that the research is affluence centred; that it is ahistoric; and that it has neglected recent developments in social theory. We comment briefly on the first two of these before moving to consider the third in more detail.

It is self-evident that much of the published research on inequalities in health is strongly affluence-centric – concerned primarily with patterns of health and illness in richer nations. The experience of the overwhelming majority of the world's population living in poorer countries is largely absent from this literature. While this is understandable, given that most of those researching in this field are based in the rich nations, it is rarely consciously acknowledged that the findings of this research are limited in this way. In fact, in most, if not all, poor nations (where overall life expectancy for both sexes is significantly lower) the gender pattern of mortality is reversed – with female rates being higher than male. The 1980s and 1990s have also seen the emergence of non-western data on gendered inequalities in morbidity and there is a growing criticism of the dominant explanatory frames for these patterns. Fuller *et al.* (1993) for example, apply the dominant (North American) social role based explanatory model to gendered patterns of health and illness in Thailand. On the basis of their work they argue that there is 'little indication in the empirical literature that explanations for the morbidity patterns observed in the US apply to other societies . . . if we are to develop viable explanations, they should be broad in scope and ideally not culture bound' (Fuller *et al.* 1993: 253).

A second important criticism of much research comparing women's and men's experience of ill health is that it is rarely located within an historical context. As Mills (1959: 145) has argued: 'every social science – or better, every well considered social study – requires an historical scope of conception and a full use of historical material'. Attention to history certainly casts the 'story' about gender inequalities in the experience of mortality between women and men in the rich nations in a different light. The historian Edward Shorter (1982), for example, reports evidence of men surviving 20 per cent to 40 per cent longer than women in prehistoric times and argues that it was not until the end of the nineteenth century, and only in the industrializing nations of Europe and North America, that women of all ages began to outlive men (Shorter 1982). As already noted, in many areas of the world today – notably parts of Africa and Asia – women still have much higher death rates than men. This historical picture is widely recognized but, although it is often accounted for with reference to the hazards of pregnancy and childbirth, there is no consensus on the interpretations of these data. Referring to the mortality patterns in the early nineteenth century, for example, Shorter comments that:

> Nothing in women's genetic make-up pre-disposed them to die more often at age thirty three of tuberculosis or typhoid than men did. It was the harsh world in which they found themselves. Women were more liable than men to die at certain ages because their lives at those ages were much harder than men's and their resistance to infection was lower.
>
> (Shorter 1982: 237)

The potential for an historical lens to greatly enhance understanding about the social causes of ill health is illustrated in the research into social class inequalities. The research of Barker and Osmond (1987), for example, which explores differences in mortality rates between three Lancashire towns in northern England, points to the salience of the socio-economic history of these areas and, in particular to the positive contemporary health legacy of past initiatives in public housing. Similarly, Phillimore (1993) argues that economic and industrial history are important in explaining differences in the mortality rates in different wards in Sunderland in the north-east of England. Similar research might illuminate aspects of gender inequalities in health. In areas where female employment rates have traditionally been higher than the national average, in Lancashire for example, patterns of mortality among women and men might differ from those in areas where women have traditionally not had paid employment. Systematic work exploring these and similar issues still remains to be done.

Neglecting theoretical developments in the social sciences

From the perspective of this chapter, the most important criticism of current research into gender inequalities in health and illness is the lack of attention directed towards theoretical developments in the social sciences since the late 1970s. The dominant approach providing the framework for research design and analysis has been, and to some extent remains, social role theory. It can be argued that the work of the American academic Constance Nathanson set the scene for much later work. In her 1970s work she presented three explanatory models to account for 'sex' differences in the experience of morbidity: '(1) women report more illness than men because it is culturally more acceptable for them to be ill; (2) the sick role is more compatible with women's other role respons-ibilities; and (3) women have more illness than men because their assigned social roles are more stressful' (Nathanson 1975: 57).

Subsequently, research in the USA and elsewhere sought to explore the relative salience for women's health of the different social roles that they 'inhabit'. Three themes can be identified in the criticisms of this dominant social role framework. First, it failed to explore in equal depth the social roles of women and men. Rather, while researchers commonly sought explanations for gender inequalities in the experience of morbidity in the different roles that women occupy, male roles were often presented uncritically. Second, the approach to social roles has been criticized for neglecting difference among women and men and similarities between them. For example, Coltrane (1994) has argued that there has been pressure on academics to publish statistically significant differences rather than similarities between women and men and that this process has tended 'to legitimate taken-for-granted assumptions about dissimilarity' (Coltrane 1994: 44).

Some of the intellectual undercurrents associated with these criticisms have begun to surface in publications and debates about the gendered patterning of health and illness. This is illustrated to some extent in a paper by Macintyre et al. (1996) in which they point to, and challenge, what could be termed a hegemonic view of gendered patterns of ill health in much of the published research to date:

> We wish to suggest that, even when one focuses on commonly used measures (such as self-assessed health, aspects of mental health or use of health services), the 'story' about gender differences in health as presented in much recent sociological and epidemiological liter-ature, has become oversimplified and that over-generalisation has become the norm with inconsistencies and complexities in patterns of gender differences in health being overlooked . . . [T]he picture of near universal female excess morbidity has tended to persist in the general literature, taking on the characteristics of a dominant scientific paradigm with anomalous or inconsistent findings not being noticed or seriously discussed.
>
> (Macintyre et al. 1996: 621 and 623)

There is an important emerging body of work which seeks to pro-blematize the concept of gender – to 'deconstruct gender aggregates', as Annandale (1998) comments. In their research on the impact of paid work on women's and men's health, for example, Emslie et al. (1999a, 1999b) have sought to separate out the relationships between health experience, gender (as a social category) and attributes associated with masculinity and femininity for both men and women – using variables that they have termed 'orientation to gender roles'. They report that after controlling for socio-demographic and occupational characteristics and orientation to gender roles, there remained a female excess for malaise symptoms; that overall, the relationship between working conditions and health experience was broadly similar for women and men; that the characteristics of paid work were a stronger predictor of health experience than family circumstances for both women and men; and that orientation to gender role (rather than gender/sex *per se*) explained a considerable proportion of the variation in psychological distress scores. They conclude that 'this suggests the importance of acknowledging the powerful constructions of male and female, masculine and feminine in our culture and the utility of exploring their associations with morbidity' (Emslie *et al.* 1999a: 44).

Researchers have also highlighted the existence and theoretical importance of potentially competing masculinities (Hearn and Collinson 1994; Sabo and Gordon 1995). In this context Annandale (1998: 141) suggests that: 'since the sociology of masculinity suggests that male experience can be as much about privation as about privilege, it might be a fruitful basis for the study of men's higher average mortality'. Some work has begun to do this. Helgeson (1995), for example, identifies three distinct elements of gender roles (role traits; gender role conflict; and beliefs about gender roles) and explores the different relationships between these and men's experience of coronary heart disease in the USA.

Work such as this draws attention to the importance of attending to the (gendered) social meanings that people attach to their 'roles' and experiences and to the likely diversity in these meanings within genders. In her early critique of research on gender inequalities in health Clarke (1983) foregrounds the salience of gendered subjectivity in relation to health when she notes that:

> illness is multifaceted and to some extent experienced differently by different people and differently by the same people at different times . . . It may be that rates of illness are different for men and women not because men and women have a different proclivity for this 'objective' phenomenon, but rather because illness means something quite different to the members of each sex.
>
> (Clarke 1983: 69 and 71)

More recently, Annandale (1998: 159) has called for future research on gender and health to move beyond its 'socially scripted' agenda 'to explore the actual experience of social roles and the meanings that they

carry for men and women'. In doing so, however, she also acknowledges the tendency for the newly emerging research tradition focusing
on masculinity to 'turn inward' and to neglect the structural factors
shaping health experiences among men and women. This neglect of the
material basis of gendered patterns of health has been highlighted by
Stacey and Thorne (1985), who argue that the social role approach

> to the analysis of gender retains its functionalist roots, emphasising
> consensus, stability and continuity . . . The notion of 'role' focuses
> attention more on individuals than on social structures, and implies
> that 'the female role' and 'the male role' are complementary (i.e.
> separate or different but equal). The terms are depoliticizing; they
> strip experience from its historical and political context and neglect
> questions of power and conflict.
>
> (Stacey and Thorne 1985: 307)

Clarke similarly criticized the neglect of questions of power in research
on gender inequalities located within a social role framework, and states
that

> The larger conceptual issue regarding gender has to do with the
> validity and efficacy of asking questions about sex differences and
> explaining these in terms of social roles . . . We are explaining a
> minuscule and contextless behaviour when the social-structural,
> cultural and economic forces which move persons dialectically are
> ignored.
>
> (Clarke 1983: 71)

Annandale (1998: 140) argues convincingly that 'conceptualising masculinity in plural terms provides a theoretical context to explore health
inequalities within men as a group, attending not just to differences,
but also to actual relations of dominance and subordination'. She recognizes, however, this will not be sufficient to extend our understanding
of inequalities in health experience between women and men. Until the
1990s, the social role tradition within gender inequalities research has
largely failed to recognize and/or attend to recent theoretical and methodological thinking within the social sciences. These developments
highlight the neglect of the potential for creative human agency despite
the lived experience of oppression and disadvantage; the notion that
individuals are not simplistically members of homogenous social groups
(defined in terms of class, ethnicity, age, ability, gender, and so on) but
rather inhabit, and negotiate, multiple social positions to which they
assign greater or lesser significance over time and place; and the recognition that these social positions reflect both social roles and social
relationships of power and control (see Giddens 1991; F. Williams 1999;

F. Williams *et al.* 1999). Although there is growing evidence that these developments are beginning to inform research on women's and men's experience of ill health, there has been an enduring tendency to look separately at structural and personal/individual influences.

Popay and her colleagues (1998) have highlighted a number of criticisms of the existing body of work on social class inequalities in health which are equally relevant to research into gender inequalities, and which resonate to some extent with the critiques discussed above. First, they argue that

> existing methods [in the dominant quantitative research] are simply not up to grasping the complexity inherent in the processes which shape health and illness [and therefore] epidemiologist's empirical investigations . . . have left them dealing with surface appearances only . . . which leaves the aetiological role of the social structure unquestioned.
>
> (Popay *et al.* 1998: 67–8)

Second, they point to the absence of concepts which allow us to better understand the relationship between 'the experience and action of individual human beings – seen potentially at least, as creative agents acting on, and shaping the world around them – and structures of power and control within which they are embedded' (Popay *et al.* 1998: 70). Third, and less importantly from the perspective of this chapter, they point to the relative absence of attention to the salience of 'historical time' and of notions of 'place' from this body of research.

Popay and her colleagues suggest that the most significant missing components of research into class inequalities in health, and we would argue also of research into gender inequalities, is attention to the theoretical framework within which research is located and to the meanings people attach to their experiences. This 'lay knowledge', they suggest, 'in narrative form could provide invaluable insights into the dynamic relationships between human agency and wider social structures that underpin inequalities in health' (Popay *et al.* 1998: 76). Before attempting to illustrate what these potential insights might be in relation to inequalities in health, we turn briefly in the next section to consider the need for greater attention to theory in the measurement of ill health in this field and then to explore in more detail the 'substance' of narratives.

Theorizing health and illness in gender inequalities research

The difficulties inherent in theorizing health and illness is a much debated topic within the social sciences (and, although it may be considered less problematic within epidemiology, similar discontent and unease at the inadequate theoretical basis for much of the measurement of health and illness is also apparent). These issues are no less relevant to research into gender inequalities in health as a paper by Macintyre *et al.* (1996) illustrates. Their analysis is based on three general measures of health status, two symptom based scales – malaise and physical symptoms – and a list of chronic or episodic conditions. The analysis also includes two different databases, but this is a complexity that will be ignored for the purposes of this discussion.

In terms of the mean number of symptoms, Macintyre *et al.* (1996) report that overall there is a consistent and significant female excess in all three of the age groups considered. They report a similar female excess for two of the age groups for the physical symptom scale and for all three age groups for the malaise scale. They then look at gender patterns across individual symptoms and find that only two of these show a significant male excess, but between six and eight out of the eighteen symptoms (depending on the age group and data set being considered) show no significant gender difference.

In contrast, in an analysis conducted by Popay *et al.* (1993) using one of the same data sets, a significant female excess was found for two different age groups for both a malaise and a physical symptom scale. These different results are probably due to the inclusion, in their analysis, of the tiredness symptom in the physical symptom scale rather than the malaise scale and broader age bands. Similarly, while Macintyre *et al.* (1996) report no significant female excess, except in the youngest age group for one data set, for the general health question and for long term illness, Blaxter (1990), using the same data but again constructing different measures with different age groups, reports significant female excesses for physical illness and disability across their longer lifespan.

The critical issue here, of course, is not which of these analyses are correct in some absolute sense, or which provide a more 'accurate' picture of some 'real' gendered pattern of ill health. Rather, the point is that much of the current literature seeks to represent and explore patterns of morbidity between women and men using measures which in large part have no theoretical basis and which can be and are changed in important ways at the 'whim' of a researcher. What, one might ask, at least from a sociological perspective, is the theoretical rationale for separating symptoms into malaise and physical? Why should tiredness be a malaise symptom rather than a physical symptom? Perhaps most importantly, what is the theoretical import of concluding that while women do have significantly higher rates of 'malaise' than men in all age groups and across all social positions (perhaps the most consistent finding from research on gendered patterns of ill health regardless of the measure of 'malaise' or psychological distress used), they do not have a consistent excess of minor 'physical' health problems?

Most of those involved in research on gender inequalities in health are aware of these problems. There are also related problems with the measurement of complex social phenomena such as work and domestic labour (Emslie *et al.* 1999a). In this context, Macintyre *et al.* (1996) argue that in the future research on 'differences' in health and illness experience between women and men should address 'the social and historical context of our observations and . . . take a more differentiated age-specific and condition specific view of "health" when examining differences between the sexes' (Macintyre *et al.* 1996: 624). We would argue that there is much analytical purchase to be gained from research which focuses on single symptoms and/or particular health problems. However, there remains a danger that research will continue to be underpinned by a medical and/or atheoretical approach to the conceptualization and operationalization of health and illness and a simplistic approach to the measurement of social position and structural dimensions. The central point is that research must be located within a theoretical framework which makes explicit the salience of a particular symptom and/or health problem to the gendering of health experience. If the measures used to explore differences in health experiences between women and men have a firmer theoretical basis then they have explanatory power over and above merely describing (contested) patterns, which still remain to be explained. In developing such a theoretical framework there is clearly a role for both qualitative and quantitative research, but it is primarily with the former that the rest of this chapter is concerned.

The substance of narratives

The representations that people give of their lived experiences have been termed 'narratives'. Some, albeit not all, qualitative research is concerned to 'capture' these representations through, for example, in-depth unstructured interviews, conversations and ethnographic fieldwork. Narratives have been called 'stories' (see e.g. Graham 1984) because they usually have 'plots', are eventful and can be full of images (Mattingley and Garro 1994). They are, however, much more than stories in the common-sense meaning of this word – that is something imagined and/or other than factual. As Mattingley and Garro note in their editorial to a special edition of *Social Science and Medicine* devoted to the narrative representation of illness and healing,

Narrative offers what is perhaps our most fundamental way to understand life in time. Through narrative we try to make sense of

how things have come to pass and how our actions and the actions
of others have helped shape our history; we try to understand who
we are becoming by reference to where we have been.

(Mattingley and Garro 1994: 771)

The contributors to that special issue explore the type of knowledge and
understanding about illness provided by narratives. In sum, Mattingley
and Garro suggest, these papers highlight how narratives about illness
give meaning to experience and can be concerned with the past and
present, and anticipate the future. They point to the social and cultural
embeddedness of narratives and the important role they play in mediating
(the sometimes contradictory) relationship between individual experience
and normative expectations. Additionally, and theoretically more significant, Somers (1994) has argued that research is revealing the substance of
narratives as central to our understanding of social action:

> Namely, that social life is storied and that narrative is an ontolo-
> gical condition of social life . . . showing us that stories guide action;
> that people construct their identities (however multiple and chang-
> ing) by locating themselves or being located within a repertoire of
> emplotted stories; that 'experience' is constituted through narratives;
> that people make sense of what has happened and is happening to
> them by attempting to assemble or in some way to integrate these
> happenings within one or more narratives; and that people are
> guided to act in certain ways and not others on the basis of the
> projections, expectations and memories derived from a multiplic-
> ity but ultimately limited repertoire of available social, public and
> cultural narratives.
>
> (Somers 1994: 614)

Life narratives, generated through qualitative research, may point up
new ways of understanding and/or interpreting gendered patterns of
health and illness because they have the potential to illuminate the relationship between gender and health experiences in ways which other
forms of 'knowing' the social world – particularly those located within
a quantitative tradition – cannot provide. First, people's accounts of
their experiences are the means by which they (re)construct their sense
of who they are in the context of the social and material world and
biographical and historical time. Narrative accounts of experience therefore illuminate the subjectively experienced relationship between identity (people's sense of who they are), agency (an individual's capacity
for action) and social structures (macro mechanisms and processes by
which power and control are socially distributed and utilized) which
impinge on the ways in which individuals negotiate/live their lives.

Second, in telling their stories, people also tell about the multiple and fluid social locations they occupy, how and why these change across time and 'place' and the salience of these for their lived experience. Third, narratives open up a window on what Finch (1989) has termed 'normative guidelines and timetables'. These are, according to Finch, the culturally transmitted sense of 'the proper thing to do' and the 'proper time to do things' which shape individual behaviour, but not in any simple way. Rather, in acting to 'mobilize obligations' in relation to caring responsibilities in Finch's study, for example, or in making sense of, and/or responding to illness more generally, people reproduce and mould these same norms and obligations in specific ways.

In a similar vein, G. H. Williams (1984, 1993) has developed the concept of 'narrative reconstruction' to capture the way in which people living with chronic illness use narrative knowledge, and actively interpret existing social norms and cultural values, to pursue a virtuous course of action in response to the consequences of illness. This analysis highlights how, in presenting and interpreting experience through narratives, we inevitably draw on shared cultural understandings. An important additional point from the perspective of this chapter is that these same 'shared cultural understandings' also shape and guide our sense of what it is to 'be' a woman and to 'be' a man. Life narratives are therefore inevitably gendered representations of experiences and meanings. But, they also provide insights into the way in which individual identity, experience and action are themselves gendered. That is, the identities people (re)construct, their life experiences, and the action they take in response to these, are shaped directly and indirectly by patriarchal structures of power and control (alongside divisions associated with social class, racism, ageism, and so on) which have both material and cultural aspects – and narratives provide one perspective on the processes involved here.

Narrative data generated through qualitative research approaches therefore provide a means for exploring a number of the issues central to our understanding of gender inequalities in ill health. In particular this type of research may offer insights into the relationship between the gendered nature of everyday life and the experience of ill health (that is the potential pathways that link the health experience of women and men with patriarchal – and other – relationships and structures of power and control). These pathways may include the gendering of social action in response to ill health (that is the relationships between the ways people respond to ill health and patriarchal – and other – structures). Narrative data may also illuminate diversity among women and men in the experience of ill health. In the next section of the chapter, we draw on published qualitative research which has generated narrative data to explore these issues in more depth. However, given that the body of qualitative research available to us is very limited the discussion must be, of necessity, tentative and can only point to the potential for further work, rather than providing definitive arguments.

Qualitative research and gender inequalities in health

Popay's (1992) study of the experience of long term tiredness among women and men provides an example of narrative based research that offers insights into pathways that could be argued to link patriarchal structures and relationships with gendered health experiences. Tiredness is a widespread symptom in the population with a consistent and significant (in both an absolute and statistical sense) female excess. In the UK national Health and Lifestyle Survey (HALS), 20 per cent of men and 30 per cent of women aged over 18 reported being 'tired all the time' (Elliott 1999). Beneath these gross figures, however, there were important variations among women and men. Among women, those with children aged between 6 and 16 were less likely to report tiredness than those with younger children, and as the number of children that a woman is caring for increases, so too does the risk that she will report being 'tired all the time'. Although a similar pattern is evident among men, the relationship is much weaker. Long term tiredness is also much more common among women, with 14 per cent of women still reporting being tired all the time in a longitudinal follow-up of the British HALS nine years after the initial survey, compared with 7 per cent of men.

Popay's study involved longitudinal unstructured interviews with parents in twenty households with dependent children in a variety of socio-economic circumstances. Tiredness was the most frequently reported health problem for both women and men (Popay 1992). However, there were two different – and strongly gendered – accounts of tiredness. In the first type of account tiredness was represented as an intermittent and/or minor event which was a normal part of daily life and no cause for concern. This was commonly provided by men in the sample and was frequently linked to demands of paid employment. In contrast, the second type of account, which was most frequently reported by women, represented tiredness as a severe, chronic and disabling condition – described in several accounts as 'total exhaustion'. This experience was reported by women across socio-economic groups and in households with different number and ages of children. Only two of the ten men included in this analysis described this type of tiredness – one in a dual career family in which the woman worked away from home, the other in his 60s and much older than the other men in the sample. Only in exceptional circumstances did this severe tiredness trigger consultation with medical care, when it was associated with other symptoms, such as faintness. Rather, it was generally presented, like the other form of tiredness, as a 'normal' part of daily life. Crucially, however, it was not linked to daily life in general but rather to daily life caring for children and others in the context of other domestic labour demands, with or without paid employment.

In these parents' accounts, therefore, the aetiological roots of prolonged severe fatigue were directly linked to the volume and type of work associated with domestic labour and caring – work normally but not exclusively done by women. But these accounts also highlight the potential aetiological role of the way in which women (and one of the two men) reporting severe fatigue responded to the demands of domestic/caring work. A prominent aspect of their narratives is the sense that 'keeping going' and succeeding in meeting what were perceived to be 'never-ending' and/or boundless demands of caring responsibilities is a central element of the 'proper thing' for mothers to do – to use the notion of normative guidelines developed by Finch (1989). This was accepted as such by most, albeit not all, of the women and the men in this study. 'Keeping going' meant, in some instances, ignoring minor ailments, doing several tasks at once, ignoring one's own needs for sleep, leisure and/or a break and juggling the competing demands of paid and domestic labour. In contrast, in men's accounts of the demands of fatherhood – even when men were the main caregivers in 'role reversal' households – there was a sense that their 'job specification' involved more clearly and narrowly delineated boundaries of responsibilities both temporally and substantively. Furthermore, in all these households, even when men were more heavily involved in the domestic and caring work than their partners, the women retained 'managerial' and supervisory responsibilities for caring and domestic labour.

These findings resonate with research in the USA by Simon (1995) on the meanings that women and men attach to work and family roles and the salience of these for gendered patterns of mental ill health. Simon uses qualitative data from follow-up interviews with women and men involved in a larger survey (albeit that these interviews did not appear to have generated narrative data, in the sense of allowing respondents to 'tell their own stories'). On the basis of this analysis she argues that gender differences in the perceived relationship between work and family roles mean that women experience more and different conflict between paid employment and parenthood than men; that women and men tend to 'blame' women who have paid employment for any marital problems that arise as a result; and that women are more likely than men to feel guilty about combining paid employment with parenthood. Additionally, mirroring some of the findings of Popay's study on the nature of the caring responsibilities that women and men describe, Simon (1995) argues that while men reported conflict between roles that was limited in scope and specific, for women the conflict was 'diffuse, non-specific and pervasive'.

Simon's study is an important illustration of the extent to which the 'shared cultural understandings' attaching to social roles are not only strongly gendered but also shared by women and men. It also points to the potential aetiological significance of these different 'meanings' for the mental health of women and men. However, the critical issue is not, as she argues, that previous research has focused exclusively on structural factors and ignored the subjective meanings women and men attach to social roles. Rather, the central problem with much research on gender inequalities is that it fails to address the theoretical and empirical linkages between structure and meaning and to consider how this iterative relationship impinges on the experience of health and illness – whether directly or through the shaping of social action. These linkages are foregrounded, albeit to a limited extent, in the accounts of prolonged tiredness reported in Popay's study. It is apparent in these accounts that at a normative level an unequal division of domestic labour is socially sanctioned and generally widely accepted by women and men – as appears to be the case in Simon's study. But the accounts of prolonged fatigue also highlight how this inequality is shaped and reinforced at a material level in terms of the differential volume and nature of the domestic and caring work that these women and men do, their differential access to material resources, and the differential constraints and opportunities offered by paid employment. From this perspective, the female excess in the experience of prolonged tiredness can be seen as arising from the interaction between material and ontological factors – that is, the material reality of caring responsibilities and the cultural centrality of these responsibilities for women's identities as mothers are interdependent.

This interaction between the material and the ontological is also captured in Graham's (1987, 1993) work on the pivotal role of 'coping' in women's conceptions of good mothering. For women to admit to not being able to cope with the emotional and physical demands of caring, according to Graham, would be equivalent to admitting to failure as a mother. Graham has focused, in particular, on the ways in which smoking behaviour among poor women can be conceptualized as a coping strategy with profound implications for health so highlighting dimensions of difference between women alongside similarities. Research has explored other 'coping strategies' among women which might 'explain' other elements of gendered health experiences. There have been studies, for example, of the ways in which women restrict their diets, walk rather than use public transport or cars, have restricted leisure activities, and reduce home heating during the day, in attempting to reconcile the demands on their time, financial resources and mental and emotional energy deriving from domestic and caring responsibilities. Despite some limited redistribution, these responsibilities are still predominantly seen to be – and are – women's.

Bendelow's (1993) qualitative study of women's and men's perceptions of the experience of pain takes these arguments about the aetiological salience of coping strategies in the context of patriarchal structures and ideology beyond the focus on women's caring responsibilities. As Bendelow notes, a consistent female excess of intermittent and chronic pain is reported in much epidemiological research. Against this backdrop she undertook a survey of women's and men's perceptions of the causes of pain and in-depth interviews exploring their experience of pain and ideas about gender differences. She reports that, in the interview, both sexes argued that women were better able to tolerate and/or cope with pain than men, and that the interviews 'revealed sophisticated explanations for this combining biological and socio-cultural perspectives' (Bendelow 1993: 290).

In summary, pain was represented in these interviewees' accounts as 'normal' for women, because of the experience of childbirth and differential socialization. In contrast, both women and men expressed the view that socialization processes actively discouraged emotional expression among boys and men, encouraging stoicism and the denial of pain. As a result, Bendelow suggests, her respondents shared the view that men would take longer to admit to pain than women. Importantly, however, respondents also felt that once men did report their pain, they were more likely than women to be taken seriously by health workers. In a related study Bendelow also found that the health workers interviewed in a study clinic believed that women were more likely than men to suffer from pain with psychogenic rather than physical origins. 'These gendered assumptions', she argues, 'may be double edged, in that the expectation of being able to 'cope' may lead to inflicting or ignoring pain [among women]' (1993: 290). In conclusion Bendelow points to the relevance of her analysis for our understanding of gender patterns of ill health and highlights the relationship between the material and the ontological:

> pain is an everyday experience linking the subjective sense of self to the perceived 'objective' reality of the world and other people. In these aspects, the gendering of culture must affect and inform the experience of pain. It is this process that is likely to hold important

clues to the well documented picture of gender inequalities in health and illness.

(Bendelow 1993: 291)

Research exploring the linkages between the ontological and material dimensions of daily life and/or social roles, the gendered ways in which people respond to the tensions between and within these, and the experience of ill health among men is particularly limited. However, there is some qualitative work exploring men's (and women's) perceptions of, and responses to, chronic and/or life-threatening illness which offers some insights into processes that may operate at a more general level. Notable here is the work of Charmaz (1995) and Gordon (1995).

Both researchers are concerned with the way in which aspects of male gender roles in contemporary western societies shape men's experience of serious illness and their responses to it. They suggest that these responses may in turn contribute to further ill health, notably psychological illness and distress. Gordon (1995) focuses on a particular disease – testicular cancer – while Charmaz (1995) is concerned more generally with the experience of chronic illness, whatever its genesis. Despite these important differences there are powerful similarities in the issues raised in these studies.

As others have shown (Zola 1966, 1973; G. H. Williams 1984; F. Williams 1999) major illness experiences, along with other significant life events such as divorce and bereavement, challenge people's sense of who they are at a normative level, as well as disrupting the material and substantive basis of daily life. Re-creating a socially acceptable and meaningful identity is a crucially important aspect of the way in which people deal or cope with life-threatening and/or chronic illness, in part by shaping the way they respond to it at a practical and psychological level. As Williams (1984, 1993) has demonstrated in his work with people with musculo-skeletal problems, in order to achieve this reconstruction people need to draw on narrative knowledge embedded in shared cultural understandings of social roles, for example, and act on the world about them, involving themselves in activities which constitute and reinforce identity. Gordon (1995) and Charmaz (1995) both highlight the ways in which men's sense of themselves as men are challenged by serious/chronic illness. As Charmaz (1995: 267) notes, 'Chronic illness can undermine all the taken for granted identities that support and sustain a man's place in the gender order including his place in the male dominance hierarchy among men . . . lessons in chronicity challenge men's assumptions about male mastery and competence'.

But these writers also both conclude that, in seeking to re-establish ontological certainty, men typically look to re-establish characteristics which are associated with traditional notions of masculinity. Gordon argues, for example, that men's verbalization of the process as one of 'fighting' cancer allows a reaffirmation of masculinity and that 'in effect they [men] arrive at a secure sense of their masculinity by defining themselves through several of the key characteristics of the traditional male sex role' (Gordon 1995: 259). Attempting to (re)involve themselves in activities that are seen to be male – for example, seeking to maintain previous levels and type of employment activity – is a central part of this process.

Charmaz (1995) and Gordon (1995) also both report some evidence of men exploring alternative responses to the disruption of serious illness – considering different 'ways of being men' – but these were most often developed alongside the pursuit of the traditional male characteristics and were limited. In Gordon's study, for example, some men noted that their cancer experience had made them more sensitive to others, but this was usually expressed as a desire to offer practical help rather than emotional support. Both authors argue that men do not handle the emotionality of their experiences well and note that men's coping strategies can also have ramifications for partners/wives. Charmaz (1995: 282) argues that women 'provide pivotal identity supports for their partners', a process which, Gordon (1995: 259) notes, can 'further polarise their [men's] relationship with women into male instrumental behaviour and female expressive behaviour'.

Both authors suggest that individual responses to one's own or partner's serious/chronic illness are strongly gendered. Comparing the responses of the men in his study and their wives, for example, Gordon argues that men typically adopt a task oriented approach to coping while women alter their emotions and mobilize family support. Charmaz, comparing the response of men and women to their own chronic illness, suggests that

> women ordinarily articulated their concerns more directly and arrived at positive conclusions more readily [than men] . . . except for those whose diseases caused severe mental impairment women showed more resiliency and resourcefulness than men in preserving aspects of self, even though women were less likely to have spouses to bolster their efforts.
>
> (Charmaz 1995: 280)

In seeking to explain these gender differences Charmaz (1995: 280) suggests that 'quite possibly, women's earlier roles and identities fostered greater adaptability to illness'. In particular she highlights as crucial differences the individualistic nature of men's responses and their focus on action as a key element of identity, compared with women's expressiveness and embeddedness in relationships. Both Charmaz and Gordon argue that men's responses to serious and/or chronic illness may exacerbate the problems associated with it and leave them vulnerable to prolonged depression. Unfortunately, neither author explores the impact on coping strategies of diversity between women (and men) in terms of childcare responsibilities and other aspects of the social and economic environment. Charmaz does, however, call for more research to take account both of this wider social context and to compare the narrative accounts of chronic illness among women and men.

Conclusion

Others have written about a contemporary backlash directed at feminist theory, analysis and praxis (see e.g. Oakley and Mitchell 1997). In some respects, a similar, not necessarily fully conscious, process is underway in relation to the academic study of gender inequalities in health. We are told that men's health problems have been neglected in the feminist flurry to identify the (arguably) unequal experience of women. Such statements, however, are clearly based on a myopic view of the field of study and, in particular, neglect the overwhelmingly male focused research on class inequalities in health. Similarly, the increasingly dominant postmodern interest in dimensions of difference – important though it has been in opening up new avenues of inquiry – is shifting attention away from the equally salient axis of structural divisions which powerfully sculpt the lives of women and men in gender differentiated ways. Interestingly, this process has parallels in other realms where, for example, it is increasingly argued that social class is no longer a salient aspect of individual identity and experience in the west (Edgell *et al.* 1995).

Notwithstanding that some 'exceptional' women and men inhabit, to a greater or less extent, the 'other's' public and domestic worlds, or that other divisions associated with class, racism, sexuality and so on divide groups of women (and men) from each other, there can be no denying the profound and enduring inequalities in the life chances of women and men. As Evans (1994), in her introduction to the reader *The Woman Question*, noted:

> Despite all these radical [social and economic] changes . . . there has been relatively little change in two important social relationships . . . the first is that of the continuing social inequality between women and men. The second sex is still precisely that: throughout the West, women have a lower level of higher and professional education than men, they are paid less, have less social power and are still assumed to have the primary . . . responsibility for the care

of children and dependent relatives. The 'new' woman remains just as much a fiction (or no doubt in some quarters a spectre) as the 'new' man . . . a second social relationship . . . remains, that between countries of the 'North' and the 'South' . . . just as social and material inequalities exist between the sexes in the 'North' so they exist and are magnified tenfold in countries in the 'South'.

(Evans 1994: 1–2)

Temporal changes in patterns of employment and family life and, as Annandale (1998) has argued, in mortality rates and the prevalence of major diseases, signal a transformation in the contours of gender inequalities. But while the morphology of gender inequalities may be transformed, all the evidence points to their continued salience. In this context, we would argue, the central question facing researchers concerned with the relationship between gender and health is how the gendering of the social, cultural, material and ontological dimensions of daily life shape women's and men's health experiences. In this chapter we have argued that our ability to answer this question has been severely hampered in the past by a failure of the research community's 'sociological imagination' (Mills 1959). This is not a narrow disciplinary point, but a comment on the poverty of social theory in research on gender inequalities in health.

We have sought to highlight three particular dimensions of the imaginative social inquiry that we believe is needed in this field in the future. First, we have suggested that there is an urgent need for more research which seeks to illuminate the relationship between health experience, identity, agency and structure – between the experience of health and ill health, people's understanding of who they are, purposeful social action, and the material aspects of their lives. Second, we have suggested, as others have (see e.g. Macintyre *et al.* 1996) that there is a need for stronger theoretical frameworks to guide future research and, in particular, the type of health outcome measures used in quantitative research. Third, we have attempted to illustrate the way in which qualitative research which is concerned to capture narrative accounts of daily life can contribute to our understanding of the nature and causes of gender inequalities in health.

The qualitative studies discussed in this chapter have very different foci. However, taken together they illuminate – albeit in a partial and opaque way – the complex relationships between identity, agency and social structures. These relationships are of central importance to our understanding of the social patterning of health and illness. Qualitative research suggests that there is both a strong normative basis – associated with patriarchal ideology – and an equally strong material basis – rooted in patriarchal structures and relationships and reflected in the way in which things are organized in the public and private spheres – shaping women's and men's daily lives, and that these have implications for the gendering of health experiences. It is not just that women and men believe that women should have primary responsibility for nurture and care, it is also that most aspects of daily life (education, paid work, the benefit structure, pensions, commerce, the organization of voluntary work, and so on) are predicated largely on the basis that women *will* care (for children, elderly and disabled relatives, neighbours). And there can be severe formal and informal penalties imposed if women fail to do so. So women's caring responsibilities are driven and shaped by both ontological and material dimensions. Women have an ontological imperative to 'care', but they develop various strategies for coping with the physical and emotional demands of caring in the context of the other calls on their time and energies. In turn, it can be argued, that these demands and coping strategies provide potential aetiological pathways to the female excess of 'minor' physical and mental ill health, such as tiredness, headaches and chronic pain. In this context, these 'health problems' can be conceptualized as health related indicators of 'oppression'.

Existing qualitative research provides relatively few insights into men's experience of health and illness and more qualitative research focusing on women and men is urgently needed. Additionally, we have not attempted to relate our arguments to gendered patterns of mortality – though we acknowledge that it would be important to do this at some stage. We would argue, however, that the work we have reviewed supports the argument that at least some elements of gender differences in health experiences are the product of the interaction between the individual pursuit of ontological stability – the (re)construction of identity – and the material conditions of daily life in the context of patriarchal structures and ideologies (cross-cut by other social divisions of class, race, age, disability, and so on). Limited though it is, this research therefore suggests that such gendered patterns are rightly viewed as inequalities – that is, patterns arising from and reflecting unequal social distributions of power and control that are amenable to change through political action.

References

Annandale, E. (1998) *The Sociology of Health and Medicine*. Cambridge: Polity Press.

Annandale, E. and Hunt, K. (1990) Masculinity, femininity and sex: an exploration of their relative contribution to explaining gender differences in health, *Sociology of Health and Illness*, 12(1): 24–46.

Arber, S. (1990) Opening the 'Black box': inequalities in women's health, in P. Abbot and G. Payne (eds) *New Directions in the Sociology of Health*. Brighton: Falmer.

Barker, D. J. P. and Osmond, C. (1987) Inequalities in health in Britain: specific explanations in three Lancashire towns, *British Medical Journal*, 294: 749–52.

Bendelow, G. (1993) Pain perceptions, emotions and gender, *Sociology of Health and Illness*, 15(3): 273–94.

Blaxter, M. (1990) *Health and Lifestyles*. London: Tavistock.

Charmaz, K. (1995) Identity dilemmas of chronically ill men, in D. Sabo and D. Gordon (eds) *Men's Health and Illness: Gender, Power and the Body*. London: Sage.

Clarke, J. (1983) Sexism, feminism and medicalism: a decade review of literature on health and illness, *Sociology of Health and Illness*, 5(1): 62–82.

Coltrane, S. (1994) Theorizing masculinities in contemporary social sciences, in H. Brod and M. Kaufman (eds) *Theorizing Masculinities*. Thousand Oaks, CA: Sage.

Edgell, S., Walklate, S. and Williams, G. (1995) *Debating the Future of the Public Sphere*. Aldershot: Avebury.

Elliott, H. (1999) Use of formal and informal care among people with prolonged fatigue: a review of the literature, *British Journal of General Practice*, (Feb.): 131–4.

Emslie, C., Hunt, K. and Macintyre, S. (1999a) Problematising gender, work and health; the relationship between gender, occupational grade, working conditions and minor morbidity in full-time bank employees, *Social Science and Medicine*, 48: 33–48.

Emslie, C., Hunt, K. and Macintyre, S. (1999b) Gender differences in minor morbidity amongst full-time employees of a British University, *Journal of Epidemiology and Community Health*, 53(8): 465–75.

Evans, M. (ed.) (1994) *The Woman Question*. London: Sage.

Finch, J. (1989) *Family Obligations and Social Change*. Cambridge: Polity Press.

Fuller, T. D., Edwards, J. N., Sermsri, S. and Vorakitphokatorn, S. (1993) Gender and health: some Asian evidence, *Journal of Health and Social Behaviour*, 34(3): 252–71.

Giddens, A. (1991) *Modernity and Self-Identity: Self and Society in the Late Modern Age*. Cambridge: Polity Press.

Gordon, D. F. (1995) Testicular cancer and masculinity, in D. Sabo and D. Gordon (eds) *Men's Health and Illness: Gender, Power and the Body*. London: Sage.

Graham, H. (1983) *Hardship and Health in Women's Lives*. London: Harvester Wheatsheaf.

Graham, H. (1984) Surveying through stories, in C. Bell and H. Roberts (eds) *Social Researching: Politics, Problems, Practice*. London: Routledge and Kegan Paul.

Graham, H. (1987) Women's smoking and family health, *Social Science and Medicine*, 25(1): 47–56.

Graham, H. (1993) *Hardship and Health in Women's Lives*. London: Harvester Wheatsheaf.

Hearn, J. and Collinson, D. (1994) Theorizing unities and differences between men and between masculinities, in H. Brod and M. Kaufman (eds) *Theorizing Masculinities*. Thousand Oaks, CA: Sage.

Helgeson, V. S. (1995) Masculinity, men's roles, and coronary heart disease, in D. Sabo and D. Gordon (eds) *Men's Health and Illness: Gender, Power and the Body*. London: Sage.

Macintyre, S., Hunt, K. and Sweeting, H. (1996) Gender differences in health: are things really as simple as they seem?, *Social Science and Medicine*, 42(4): 617–42.

Macintyre, S., Ford, G. and Hunt, K. (1999) Do women 'over-report' morbidity? Men's and women's responses to structured prompting on a standard question on long standing illness, *Social Science and Medicine*, 48(1): 89–98.

Mattingley, C. and Garro, L. C. (eds) (1994) Narrative representations of illness and healing, special issue of *Social Science and Medicine*, 38(6): 771–4.

Mills, C. W. (1959) *The Sociological Imagination*. New York: Oxford University Press.

Nathanson, C. A. (1975) Illness and the feminine role: a theoretical review, *Social Science and Medicine*, 9(2): 57–62.

Oakley, A. and Mitchell, J. (eds) (1997) *Who's Afraid of Feminism? Seeing Through the Backlash*. London: Hamish Hamilton.

Phillimore, P. (1993) How do places shape health? Rethinking locality and lifestyle in North East England, in S. Platt, H. Thomas, S. Scott and G. Williams (eds) *Locating Health: Sociological and Historical Explorations*. Aldershot: Avebury.

Popay, J. (1992) 'My health is all right, but I'm just tired all the time': women's experience of ill health, in H. Roberts (eds) *Women's Health Matters*. London: Routledge.

Popay, J., Bartley, M. and Owen, C. (1993) Gender inequalities in health: social position, affective disorders and minor physical morbidity, *Social Science and Medicine*, 36(1): 21–32.

Popay, J., Williams, G., Thomas, C. and Gatrell, A. (1998) Theorising inequalities in health: the place of lay knowledge, *Sociology of Health and Illness*, 20(5): 619–44.

Rosser, S. V. (1994) *Women's Health: Missing from US Medicine*. Bloomington, IN: Indiana University Press.

Sabo, D. and Gordon, D. (eds) (1995) *Men's Health and Illness: Gender, Power and the Body*. London: Sage.

Shorter, E. (1982) *A History of Women's Bodies*. London: Allen Lane.

Simon, R. W. (1995) Gender, multiple roles, role meaning, and mental health, *Journal of Health and Social Behaviour*, 36: 182–94.

Somers, M. R. (1994) The narrative constitution of identity: a relational and network approach, *Theory and Society*, 23: 605–49.

Stacey, J. and Thorne, B. (1985) The missing feminist revolution in sociology, *Social Problems*, 32(4): 301–16.

Verbrugge, L. (1977a) Females and illness: recent trends in sex differences in the United States, *Journal of Health and Social Behaviour*, 17: 387–403.

Verbrugge, L. (1977b) Sex differences in morbidity and mortality in the United States, *Social Biology*, 23: 275–96.

Williams, F. (1999) Exploring links between old and new paradigm: a critical review, in F. Williams, J. Popay and A. Oakley (eds) *Welfare Research: A Critical Review*. London: UCL Press.

Williams, F., Popay, J. and Oakley, A. (eds) (1999) *Welfare Research: A Critical Review*. London: UCL Press.

Williams, G. H. (1984) The genesis of chronic illness: narrative reconstruction, *Sociology of Health and Illness*, 6: 175–200.

Williams, G. H. (1993) Chronic illness and the pursuit of virtue in everyday life, in A. Radley (ed.) *Worlds of Illness: Cultural and Biographical Perspectives on Health and Disease*. London: Routledge.

Zola, I. (1966) Culture and symptoms: an analysis of patients presenting complaints, *American Sociological Review*, 31: 615–30.

Zola, I. (1973) Pathways to the doctor – from person to patient, *Social Science and Medicine*, 7: 677–89.

four

Socio-economic change and inequalities in men and women's health in the UK

Hilary Graham

Introduction

Social class is 'written on the body': it is inscribed in our experiences of health and our chances of premature death. The invariable pattern, across time and between societies, is one in which men and women in higher socio-economic groups enjoy better health across longer lives than those in lower socio-economic groups. These inequalities in health are persisting – and in some cases are widening – in the context of rapid economic and social change. In the UK, for example, the rapid decline in manual occupations and the growth of more flexible employment contracts has brought with it greater job insecurity and unemployment. At the same time, men and women are reshaping their domestic lives, with more moving into and out of cohabitation and marriage. Changes in employment and household patterns are fuelling a wider process of socio-economic polarization. During the 1980s and 1990s greater prosperity for the majority has been at the cost of poverty for an increasing minority.

This chapter focuses on the UK, as a case study through which to turn the spotlight on socio-economic inequalities in health among men and women and the wider inequalities in life chances and living standards which underlie them. The first section of the chapter is concerned with the socio-economic patterning of men's and women's health revealed in UK data. The section briefly describes the health gradients and the material, psychosocial and behavioural factors which are seen to contribute to them and then looks at UK research on how these risk factors cluster together and accumulate across an individual's life, with low socio-economic status linked to a higher concentration and accumulation of risks. The second section of the chapter turns from inequalities in health to inequalities in wealth. It focuses on changes in the distribution of income and living standards in the UK which have particular implications for socio-economic inequalities in health. It discusses the increase in poverty and the shift in its burden down the lifecourse from older people to children and the lone mothers who care for them within a socio-economic structure in which inequalities between households have widened substantially.

In turning the spotlight on socio-economic stratification and socio-economic change, the chapter inevitably places other aspects of inequality in shadow. Age, ethnicity and sexuality, as well as gender, mediate the influence of socio-economic position on health. Socio-economic inequality, and its intersection with gender, therefore provides only a starting point for an analysis of how socio-economic change is structured into individual health. The focus on how health is framed by socio-economic circumstances also means that the chapter gives less attention to how individuals achieve agency 'in and against' these circumstances. However, the evidence it presents provides a corrective to perspectives on late modernity which suggest that the class based inequalities which have long characterized the UK are giving way to individually fashioned identities. Many men and women may, as sociological accounts have argued, be engaged in a reflexive and lifelong 'project of the self' (Giddens 1991). But increasing poverty and social polarization mean that the opportunity to participate in such projects is unequally distributed, with an increasing proportion of the population denied access to the lifestyles and life choices that the majority take for granted.

The chapter's focus on socio-economic inequalities is grounded in two fields of research: social policy and social epidemiology. Social policy research records what social change is doing to people's socio-economic circumstances, while social epidemiology is concerned with what their socio-economic circumstances are doing to their health. In their different ways, researchers in both disciplines map the pathways which run between the structure of society and the welfare of individuals. Researchers in social policy and social epidemiology share, too, a recognition of the difficulty of proving cause and effect, of demonstrating that structural factors have health outcomes. Demonstrating the health effects of changes in these structural influences is an even more complex methodological and theoretical task.

The task is complex partly because of the limitations of conventional measures of socio-economic position. In the UK, occupation and employment status have been and remain the primary measures of an individual's social class or socio-economic status (Rose and O'Reilly 1997). But, as in other countries, there are marked gender differences in employment status, with women more likely than men to be outside the labour market and in part-time employment. There is also a socio-economic gradient in full-time employment, with the proportion of men and women in full-time jobs rising with occupational social class (Office for National Statistics (ONS) 1998). Exposure to occupation related influences on health is therefore likely to be greater among men than women, and among those higher up rather than lower down the class ladder. As a result, analyses of socio-economic differences in health which are based on occupation are not, as Hunt and Macintyre (in press) put it, 'comparing like with like'. Demonstrating causal connections between socio-economic exposure and health effects is difficult, too, because an individual's health is shaped by long term processes which may be evident only when they materialize as symptoms: whether as self-defined ill health or as clinically validated indicators of disease. Further, there are likely to be time lags, of variable duration, between exposure to the cause and evidence of the effect, during which time other mediating factors may have altered the progress of the disease.

For these reasons, the chapter has a modest agenda. It seeks to highlight, first, the systematic way in which men's and women's health is shaped by socio-economic circumstances and trajectories, and second, how these socio-economic circumstances and trajectories are polarizing as the result of broader social trends.

Socio-economic inequalities in health

Patterns and trends

Socio-economic differentials in mortality have been recorded since the mid-eighteenth century (Woods and Williams 1995). By the mid-nineteenth century, these differentials were being systematically recorded in public surveys of Britain's new industrial cities (Whitehead 1997). In Liverpool in the 1840s, for example, the average age of death was 35 for the gentry and professional people, 22 for tradesmen and 15 for labourers (Whitehead 1997). This was the epidemiological period in which infectious diseases were the major causes of death. Today, the UK, like other western societies, has made the transition to a postindustrial society in which chronic diseases like coronary heart disease, stroke and cancer dominate the mortality statistics. These diseases have different specific causes, both from each other and from the killer diseases of the nineteenth century. But they share a common socio-economic profile.

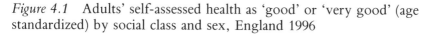

Figure 4.1 Adults' self-assessed health as 'good' or 'very good' (age standardized) by social class and sex, England 1996

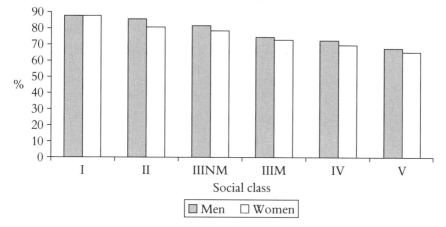

Source: Prescott-Clarke and Primatesta 1998: Table 5.14

Consistent gradients are found for most major causes of death, including lung cancer, respiratory disease, heart disease and stroke (Smith and Harding 1997). Similar gradients are evident in self-reported health (Prescott-Clarke and Primatesta 1998; ONS 1998).

While the historical focus has been on the socio-economic gradients in men's health, contemporary evidence reveals comparable differentials among women. The (limited) evidence also suggests that socio-economic status makes an important contribution to ethnic variations in health among men and women. It demonstrates, too, the limitations of traditional indicators, like occupation and housing tenure, for measuring, and for controlling the effects of, socio-economic status in different ethnic groups (Nazroo 1997).

Figures 4.1 and 4.2 describe the socio-economic gradient in men and women's health, as revealed in two measures of health status: self-assessed health and mortality. Figure 4.1 maps the proportion of men and women describing their health as 'very good' or 'good' in the Health Survey for England, which uses a measure of social class based on own occupation (Prescott-Clarke and Primatesta 1998). Figure 4.2 is based on the Office for National Statistics Longitudinal Study and classifies women's social class by the occupation of their (male) partners (Smith and Harding 1997). The gradients in mortality tend to be less steep for women but, as among men, higher socio-economic status protects women against the risk of ill health, while lower socio-economic status increases their chances of disease, disability and premature death.

Figure 4.2 Age standardized death rates per 100,000 people by social class, men and women aged 35–64, England and Wales 1980–92

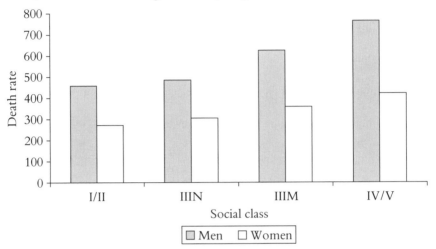

Note: Women are classified by partner's occupational details or, if absent, by their own
Source: 1971 LS Cohort, England and Wales described in Smith and Harding 1997: Tables 11.4 and 11.7

Compared to men and women in social class I, men and women in social class V have death rates which are respectively 1.7 and 1.5 times higher, while the proportion of men and women in good or very good health is around 30 per cent lower at the bottom of the class ladder than at the top.

The socio-economic differentials in health captured in Figures 4.1 and 4.2 are evident using different indicators of socio-economic position, including parental social class, education, income, housing tenure and car ownership (Filakti and Fox 1995; Smith and Harding 1997; Davey Smith *et al.* 1998). There are, of course, strong associations between these different measures of socio-economic status: staying on at school and gaining qualifications anticipates a career marked out by employment in secure and high paid non-manual occupations, which in turn provides the longer term income needed to buy a home and own a car. This suggests that the different measures are indices of an individual's socio-economic experience over the lifecourse, with parental social class indicating where a person comes from, education signalling where the person is going, and occupation and tenure marking the class of destination.

These different measures of lifetime socio-economic status not only produce pronounced class differences in health, but also suggest that the position of those in poorer circumstances has worsened relative to those in more advantaged socio-economic groups since the 1970s. Mortality provides one example. While death rates have fallen for men and women in all social classes, class differences in mortality have widened (Drever and Bunting 1997). Widening class differences in male mortality reflect widening differentials in major causes of death, including coronary heart disease, stroke, lung cancer and suicide. Among women, class differences in the risks of dying from lung cancer have also increased since the 1970s. Since the early 1980s, a steepening of the class gradient in mortality from heart disease and a flattening of the positive gradient in breast cancer mortality have also contributed to a widening of socio-economic mortality differentials among women (Drever and Bunting 1997; Harding *et al.* 1997).

How can the persistent and widening socio-economic differentials in health be explained? One possibility is that there is nothing to be explained: that the gradients are an artefact, produced through flaws in the measurement of socio-economic status and health and in the statistical analyses of their relationship. It is now generally accepted that statistical inaccuracies can not explain the consistency and magnitude of the class gradient (Davey Smith *et al.* 1994). An alternative explanation suggests that the gradient is the outcome of health related mobility, in which healthier people climb up the class ladder, while those in poorer health slip down. However, while health status influences subsequent social mobility, the evidence suggests that its scale is insufficient to explain the overall socio-economic gradients in health (Power *et al.* 1996).

With neither statistical errors nor social mobility making a major contribution to health inequalities, the search for causes has focused on factors which run back to and from the broader structure of society. However, health outcomes are not easily tracked to their class origins. Both an individual's health and the class relationships in which they experience it are dynamic, with changes reflecting longer term processes which are hard to detect through the research designs currently available. Detection tends to be easier at the individual rather than structural level: at the point at which the underlying processes manifest themselves in people's home and work environments and in their daily habits and routines. As a result, studies have revealed considerably more about factors which are proximate (close) to the individual than about factors which are proximate to the social structure.

Constrained by these limitations, researchers have worked to identify the individual-level factors which link socio-economic status and health status. Attention has focused on three sets of factors: material, psychosocial and behavioural. Material factors include the physical environment of the home, neighbourhood and workplace, together with living standards secured through earnings, benefits and other income. Psychosocial factors include the life events and chronic difficulties which make demands that are hard to meet and the social networks and confiding relationships which can support people through them. Among the behavioural factors, diet, cigarette smoking and recreational exercise have been singled out for their contribution to the socio-economic gradient. The contribution of these factors to the socio-economic gradient in health obviously varies between different dimensions of health. Material factors figure more strongly than psychosocial factors in relation to causes of death like accidental injuries and respiratory disease, while both the material and psychosocial environments are implicated in the aetiology of many psychological illnesses.

Gender, as well as socio-economic position, mediates exposure to material, psychosocial and behavioural risks. For example, men have traditionally been more exposed to the industrial injuries associated with skilled manual work (in mining, engineering and construction, for example). Men also led the way into habits like cigarette smoking at a time when it symbolized affluence and high class living, and men still have higher rates of alcohol consumption: two behavioural factors seen as contributing to the male excess of mortality from lung cancer and coronary heart disease. Conversely, women are more likely to experience the disadvantages identified as contributing to affective disorders: a poor home environment, with heavy childcare responsibilities and low levels of social support (Brown and Harris 1978; Elliot and Huppert 1991; Macran *et al.* 1996). Reviewing the evidence on these divergent gender patterns, it has been suggested that women's disadvantaged position at home and in the labour market may hold the key to understanding both women's lower rates of mortality and their higher rates of morbidity from poor mental health and particularly from anxiety and depressive disorders (Johanasson 1991; Popay *et al.* 1993; Macintyre and Hunt 1997).

Material, psychosocial and behavioural risk factors – among both men and women – tend to cluster together. Individuals exposed to material disadvantage are more likely to be disadvantaged with respect to their psychosocial environment and their health behaviour, while individuals protected from material hazards are more likely to have a protected and protective psychosocial environment and to engage in health promoting behaviours. Proximate influences not only cluster together, but also accumulate together. Children born into material disadvantage are exposed to more material, psychosocial and behavioural risk factors across their (shorter and less healthy) lives than children born into material advantage.

It is the clustered and culminative nature of disadvantage – material, psychosocial and behavioural – which is seen to produce and perpetuate

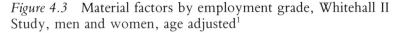

Figure 4.3 Material factors by employment grade, Whitehall II Study, men and women, age adjusted[1]

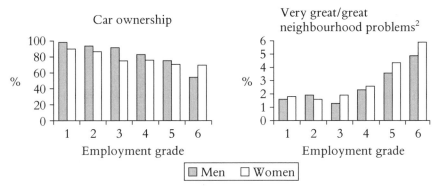

Notes
1 N = approx. 9000; tests for trend within sex by grade significant at p < 0.001 for men and women
2 Neighbourhood problems as measured by answers to the question 'To what extent do you have problems with the neighbourhood you live in (e.g. noise, unsafe streets, few local facilities)?', using a five-point scale (very great, great, some, slight and little)
Source: Whitehall II, unpublished data

inequalities in men's and women's health. Research which addresses these key dimensions of class related exposure is discussed in more detail in the two subsections below.

The clustering of material, psychosocial and behavioural risks

Socio-economic gradients in exposure to material, psychosocial and behavioural risks have been consistently found in population surveys and in surveys of specific subgroups, like the Whitehall II Study of civil servants. Civil service grade provides a finely graduated measure of socio-economic status within a relatively privileged section of the working population. Clear socio-economic differentials in health are nonetheless produced among both men and women, as measured by height, body mass index, obesity, hypertension and self-reported health (Marmot and Davey Smith 1997; Marmot *et al.* 1997).

Socio-economic gradients in individual level influences are also strongly in evidence, with broadly similar gradients among both men and women. As Figure 4.3 describes, access to material resources, proxied by car ownership, and exposure to material problems, measured by neighbourhood environment, is related to civil service grade. Psychosocial risks and resources are similarly patterned by employment

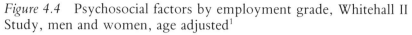

Figure 4.4 Psychosocial factors by employment grade, Whitehall II Study, men and women, age adjusted[1]

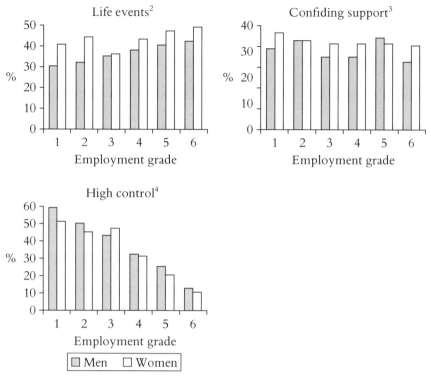

Notes
1 All analyses: N = approx. 9000; test for trend within sex by grade significant at $p < 0.001$ for men and women
2 Life events = two or more major life events
3 Confiding support = confiding support from closest person
4 High control = high control of pace and content of paid work
Source: Marmot and Davey Smith 1997: Table 3

grade (Figure 4.4). Exposure to life events among men is inversely related to civil service grade, with rates of exposure in both sexes rising as employment grade falls. Poor working conditions, as measured by low control over the pace and content of work, are also related to low employment grade. Conversely, men and women in higher grades are significantly more likely to have access to a confiding relationship and to have high control at work. Health related behaviours display a similar socio-economic profile (Figure 4.5). Among both men and women, those in the lowest grade are most likely to smoke cigarettes and least

Figure 4.5   Behavioural factors by employment grade, Whitehall II Study, men and women, age adjusted[1]

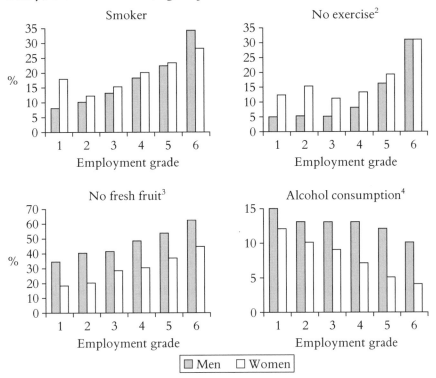

Notes
1 All analyses: N = approx. 9000; test for trend within sex by grade significant at p < 0.001 for men and women
2 No exercise = no moderate or vigorous exercise
3 No fresh fruit = fresh fruit less than daily
4 Alcohol consumption = mean units of alcohol in last seven days
Source: Marmot and Davey Smith 1997: Table 2

likely either to be taking exercise or have diets high in recommended nutrients, like fresh fruit. Alcohol consumption, however, displays a different pattern, with higher mean consumption associated with higher employment grade for both women and men. The positive socio-economic gradient in alcohol consumption is also evident in national surveys (Colhoun and Prescott-Clarke 1996; ONS 1998). These surveys point to other socio-economic differences in alcohol consumption. While affluence is associated with higher consumption, the experience of being drunk and of problem drinking is more strongly associated with deprivation.

As Figures 4.3 to 4.5 suggest, individuals' access to health promoting environments and lifestyles is strongly patterned by their socio-economic position. However, the socio-economic patterning of health risks and resources is not identical for men and women. The most striking example is cigarette smoking, where the socio-economic gradient is reversed for women in the highest employment grade (Figure 4.5). Smoking prevalence in this group is 1.5 times higher than in the grade below. Women at the top of the civil service hierarchy also have the highest rates of alcohol consumption and, unlike their male counterparts, do not have the highest rates of leisure time exercise. These divergent lifestyles may reflect, as Marmot and Davey Smith (1997) suggest, the unique pressures on women working in high grades in the civil service. They may also reflect, and interact with, other differences between men and women in senior management. For example, other studies have found gender differences in socio-economic background and household patterns of those who reach the higher grades in their organization, with women more likely to have a university degree, less likely to be married and less likely to have children than men (Emslie *et al.* 1999a, 1999b). Differences in socio-economic background and home circumstances also go some way to explaining why women employers and managers are more likely to be smokers than women in other non-manual occupations (Graham and Hunt 1994; Burrows and Nettleton 1997).

Describing the socio-economic patterning of material, psychosocial and behavioural factors among men and women is an important first stage in explaining health inequalities. But it does not, of course, demonstrate their contribution to the socio-economic gradient in health. Establishing their contribution is complicated by the fact that their influence is likely to vary between health outcomes: cigarette smoking, for example, figures more prominently than low control at work in explanations of lung cancer. Nonetheless, research is beginning to disentangle, and to quantify, the contribution of material, psychosocial and behavioural factors.

With respect to the material environment, exposure to persistent poverty is more harmful than the experience of occasional poverty (Benzeval 1998a). Studies have found large inequalities in physical and psychological health by income and by living standards, after controlling for other dimensions of socio-economic disadvantage, like education, occupation and marital status (Stronks *et al.* 1998; Weich and Lewis 1998).

With respect to the psychosocial environment, again there is evidence of its contribution to socio-economic inequalities in physical and psychological health. The Whitehall II Study has highlighted the importance of psychosocial work conditions, and low control in particular, to coronary heart disease risk. The experience of low control at work has been found to increase coronary heart disease risk independently of socio-economic status (as measured by employment grade) and other socio-economic related exposures, including social support (Marmot *et al.* 1997). In studies concerned with psychological health, however, social support has been found to play a larger role in mediating the effects of material disadvantage. A study which tested the effects of material deprivation (enforced absence of one or more basic necessities) and lack of social support (emotional and practical) on psychological health found that material deprivation was the more important influence. However, access to social support moderated this influence. Low social support had a more negative effect on the psychological health of those living in poverty, and poverty had its most substantial effects on the psychological well-being of those who had limited access to social support (Whelan 1993).

With respect to behavioural factors, an early estimate of the behavioural contribution to health inequalities was provided by the Whitehall I Study. Socio-economic differences in behavioural risk factors were estimated to account for one third of the gradient in the relative risk of death from coronary heart disease (Marmot *et al.* 1984). More recent studies have estimated that between 10 and 30 per cent of the class differential in health may be explained by class differentials in health related behaviour (Lantz et al. 1998; Stronks 1997). However, because individual behaviour can be measured with greater precision than the material and social environment, estimates of its contribution to the socio-economic gradient may be inflated (Phillips and Davey Smith 1991).

To date, gender has not been a major focus of epidemiological studies seeking to access the contribution of material, psychosocial and behavioural factors to socio-economic inequalities in health. Little is yet known about the ways in which gender, with and through other dimensions of inequality, mediates men and women's exposure to material, psychosocial and behavioural influences. What is known and recognized, however, is that women are more likely than men both to be poor and to be responsible for maintaining the material and psychosocial environment of the home and the well-being of those who live there. Men are over-represented in higher income households, while women (and children) are at greater risk of living in low income households, with limited access to material and psychosocial resources. They are also more likely to be restricted to, and to work within, these disadvantaged environments. It is estimated that 40 per cent of women in Britain spend upwards of 50 hours a week caring for members of their household (Corti and Dex 1995). The patterns of work among fathers and mothers provide one illustration of the extent to which women (still) care for the family.

In two parent households, less than 1 per cent of fathers 'look after the home' as their main economic activity and over 80 per cent are in full-time paid employment. Among mothers with dependent children, 30 per cent are engaged in home and family care and only 20 per cent are working full time (Benzeval 1998b).

Studies of women's experiences of caring on a low income have described how shortage of money restricts their access to social support – and how, without the material support of family and friends, it is hard (if not impossible) to feed the family and meet other health needs without going into debt (Kempson *et al.* 1994; Dennehy 1998). Low income and limited support combine to force mothers to rely on behaviours which compromise health in the struggle for financial survival. While seeking to protect the food budget, and children's food in particular, it is also the target for day-to-day economies and the reserve fund for unexpected emergencies. This is because food is both the largest single item of spending in low income households and the one over which women exercise most direct control. Particularly for women who do not live within walking distance of relatives able and willing to provide meals on a regular basis, foods which they recognize are essential elements of their children's diet – like fresh fruit – are either strictly rationed, or off the menu (Kempson *et al.* 1994; Graham 1998).

As the evidence reviewed in this section suggests, the distribution of positive and negative influences on health is patterned by socio-economic status and gender. In different ways and to varying degrees, access to health promoting material, psychosocial and behavioural resources increases in line with increasing socio-economic status, for both men and women. Conversely, the rate of exposure to material, psychosocial and behavioural risks increases with declining socio-economic status. But it is not only the combined effects of access and exposure which have been highlighted in epidemiological studies. The accumulation, as well as the combination, of risks is seen to play a central part in the pathways which link social class to individual health.

Culminative exposure to material, psychosocial and behavioural risks

The way in which access to resources and exposure to risks combine can be captured in cross-sectional surveys, where measures are taken at one point in time. However, to track how these resources and risks accumulate over the lifecourse requires longitudinal studies, where measures are taken from the same population at different points in time. Birth cohort studies, which follow a cohort of babies into childhood and adulthood, are the research design of choice. They enable both the process of accumulation and its health effects to be monitored. The

Figure 4.6   Exposure to material, psychosocial and behavioural risks in childhood by social class at birth, National Child Development Study

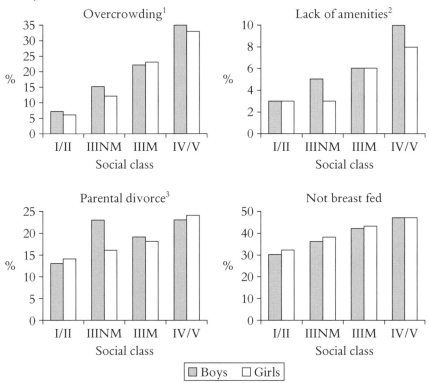

Notes
1 Overcrowding = more than one person per room
2 Lack of amenities = lacking or sharing bathroom, toilet or hot water supply with another household
3 Parental divorce = before child was 16 years old
Source: Power and Matthews 1997: Tables 3 and 5

British birth cohort studies, and the 1958 National Child Development Study in particular, have recorded how exposure to disadvantage 'casts long shadows forward', both over a person's future socio-economic status and future health.

The long shadows of disadvantage mean that children born into poorer circumstances accumulate more material, psychosocial and behavioural risks (Figure 4.6). In the 1958 cohort study, girls and boys born into social class IV and V (based on their father's occupation) were much more likely to grow up in overcrowded homes lacking household

Figure 4.7 Exposure to a poor psychosocial environment at age 33 by social class at birth, National Child Development Study

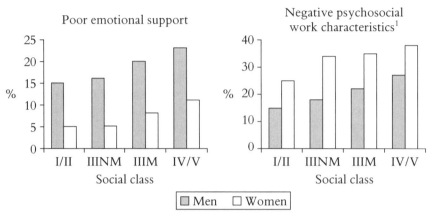

amenities than those in higher social classes. The psychosocial environment of childhood was similarly patterned by social class, with a socio-economic gradient in exposure to such life events as the divorce of one's parents. Parental health related behaviours, such as breast feeding, were also related to childhood social class.

The process of differential accumulation of risks continued into adulthood. By the time the 1958 birth cohort reached the age of 33 (in 1991), there were sharp socio-economic gradients by father's social class in the proportions of women and men living with material disadvantage (in rented housing, on means-tested benefits, having no savings and having debts). There were also socio-economic differences in the psychosocial environment (lacking emotional and practical support, doing work characterized by low control and monotony, perceiving one's job as insecure). Gender mediated these socio-economic differences in psychosocial factors (Figure 4.7). Women were less likely to experience poor social support than men at each level of the class hierarchy. Conversely, women's main jobs (paid or unpaid) were characterized by more negative psychosocial characteristics. Only among women from social class I/II did the proportion of women with negatively perceived job characteristics fall below one-third (to 25 per cent). Among men, it was only among those with fathers in social class IV/V that the proportion reached this level.

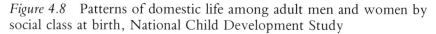

Figure 4.8   Patterns of domestic life among adult men and women by social class at birth, National Child Development Study

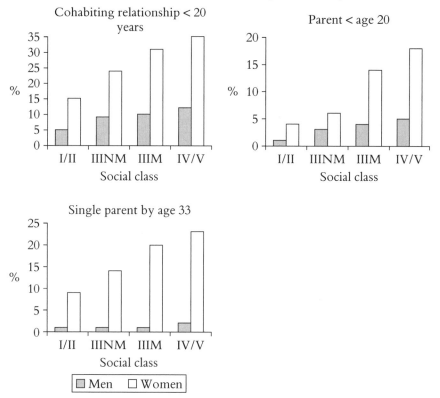

Source: Power and Matthews 1997: Table 5

With respect to behavioural factors, the consistent socio-economic gradient again displayed gender differences. For example, men in each class group reported poorer diets than women (Power and Matthews 1997).

Framing the gendered socio-economic gradients captured in Figure 4.7 are men and women's different positions within the structures of inequality into which they are born. Gender makes a difference to how men and women live their class positions and class makes a difference to how they live their gender (Skeggs 1997). A glimpse into these interlocking processes is provided in Figure 4.8, which describes the patterns of domestic life among young adults in the 1990s. Again, it is based on the 1958 cohort study and again men and women are classified by their social class (based on father's occupation) at birth.

As Figure 4.8 suggests, social class expresses itself in a gendered form. Particularly striking is the way in which both gender and class mediated the investments which the 1958 cohort made in their domestic lives. In early adulthood, it was women, and working class women in particular, who invested in identities built around partners and children. By the age of 20, 1 in 20 men born into the highest social class group were in a cohabiting relationship and 1 in 100 were fathers. Among women in the lowest social class group, 1 in 3 were cohabiting and 1 in 6 were mothers by this age. These gendered class patterns continue into later adulthood. At the age of 33, lone fatherhood was both an unusual role for men and one without a marked class gradient: 1 per cent of men from social class I/II and 2 per cent of men from social class IV/V were single parents. Among women, lone parenthood was both more common and was strongly class related. At the age of 33, 9 per cent of women born to fathers in social class I/II were lone mothers, a proportion rising to 23 per cent among women born into families in social class IV/V. In the UK, lone parenthood – for women if not for men – is strongly associated with low income, and with dependency on means-tested benefits in particular (see pp. 109–10).

Longitudinal studies like the 1958 birth cohort study not only have revealed how childhood disadvantage increases the risk of disadvantage across the lifecourse, but also have described the long shadow that lifecourse disadvantage casts over health. Socio-economic circumstances at each stage of childhood and early adolescence are related to health in adult life (Power *et al.* 1991; Power and Matthews 1997). For example, a Scottish cohort study of employed men found marked differences in the mortality rates of men in manual and non-manual occupations, with the mortality risk increasing in line with the length of time spent in a manual job (Davey Smith *et al.* 1997).

In analysing the health effects of exposure to disadvantage, attention has focused on the question of whether there are periods of life which have particularly powerful effects on subsequent health (Kuh and Ben-Shlomo 1997). For example, is exposure to risks in early life more detrimental to adult health than exposures in later childhood and adulthood? An important seam of research has focused on in-utero exposures, hypothesizing that under-nutrition in pregnancy 'programmes' an individual's susceptibility to disease in adulthood (Barker 1998). The range of diseases include causes of mortality like coronary heart disease, stroke and chronic bronchitis which make a significant contribution to the socio-economic gradient in men and women's health. Exposure to poor material conditions in infancy and childhood has also been identified as having a long term effect on adult health, independent of adult socio-economic status (Lundberg 1991; Power 1991; Mheen 1998). While these findings point to the need to protect the living standards of (future) mothers and children, households with children have found themselves at the sharp end of rising poverty and increasing social polarization.

Widening socio-economic inequalities

Patterns and trends

Health inequalities in Britain have been persisting and widening against a backdrop of increasing national prosperity. Average real incomes (calculated to allow for inflation) grew by about 40 per cent between the late 1970s and the mid-1990s, and an increasing proportion of the population now both own their home and have access to a car (Hills 1997; ONS 1998). However, the steady improvement in living standards recorded in national data masks more complex economic and social changes.

Britain's economic base has shifted away from the traditional manufacturing industries which provided full-time jobs to manual workers to service sector employment characterized by more flexible and less secure jobs. An increase in unemployment, and in male unemployment in particular, has been one outcome of this process. Male unemployment climbed from under 4 per cent in the early 1970s to 14 per cent in the mid-1990s. Changes in the structure of employment have coincided with changes in housing tenure and family structure. In 1950, 70 per cent of households rented their home; in the late 1990s nearly 80 per cent were owner-occupiers (ONS 1998). Household patterns have also changed radically across this period. In the 1950s and 1960s, men and women across the class spectrum followed a similar route through adult life. The vast majority married in their early 20s, had their first baby within three years of marriage and remained married until separated by death (Kiernan 1989). In the 1990s men and women are fashioning more diverse and dynamic household patterns as they move through adulthood and into old age. These new pathways are marked out by an increase in single adult households, in cohabitation, in births outside marriage and in separation, divorce and remarriage.

One result of these trends is a rapid growth in the number of one parent families, the vast majority of which are headed by women. In 1971, approximately one in thirteen (8 per cent) of all households with dependent children was headed by a lone mother. By the mid-1990s, it was one in five (20 per cent) (Haskey 1998). Since the late 1980s, it is the increase in single (never married) lone mothers which has fuelled the upward trend in the number of one parent families. Lone mothers in the UK are more disadvantaged than in other western countries, with a smaller proportion in employment and higher proportion in poverty (Bradshaw 1996). However, in countries like Sweden, where lone mothers have previously had high employment levels and low poverty rates, there has been a deterioration in their socio-economic circumstances through the 1980s and 1990s (Burstrom *et al.* in press). Trends in the UK may therefore be prefiguring changes elsewhere in Europe.

Trends in employment, housing tenure and household composition are combining in ways which are reshaping the social landscape of Britain. Among the features of the new landscape which are likely to affect the socio-economic patterning of men and women's health are the increase in poverty and childhood poverty and the wider process of socio-economic polarization of which the increase in poverty is part.

Increasing poverty and childhood poverty

Following the deep and widespread poverty of the 1930s, the UK experienced a long period of narrowing income differentials. Between 1939 and 1976, differences in the real incomes – and therefore the living standards – of rich and poor households narrowed. In other words, poorer households were able to afford more of the resources that better-off households took for granted. From the mid-1970s, the trend toward greater income inequality went into reverse (Goodman *et al.* 1997). Across the next two decades, inequalities in living standards in the UK increased at a pace and to a scale unmatched in Europe.

While better-off households enjoyed rising living standards, the number of households on low incomes increased. Through the 1980s and early 1990s, the proportion of the population living in households with incomes below the European Union (EU) decency threshold rose sharply. The threshold is represented by a household income below half the average for all households, adjusted for size and composition. This relative poverty line defines as poor those who experience an enforced lack of socially defined necessities. Figure 4.9 plots the proportion of the UK population living in households below the EU decency threshold. As it indicates, 7 per cent were in poverty in the mid-1970s; by the early 1990s, nearly a quarter (24 per cent) of the population were living in households with incomes less than half the national average (after housing costs). While the scale of poverty has fallen slightly since then, to 23 per cent in 1994/5, it is still three times higher than it was two decades earlier (Hills 1997).

The increased burden of poverty has not been equally shared by all age and household groups. At a time when the cohort studies have been highlighting the long term effects of childhood disadvantage on health and socio-economic status, there has been a shift in the risk of poverty

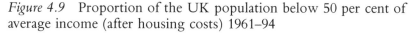

Figure 4.9 Proportion of the UK population below 50 per cent of average income (after housing costs) 1961–94

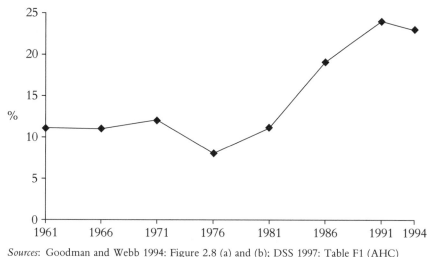

Sources: Goodman and Webb 1994: Figure 2.8 (a) and (b); DSS 1997: Table F1 (AHC)

down the lifecourse. Through the 1980s and early 1990s, the number of pensioners in the poorest groups fell, while the risks of poverty increased for children. In 1975, there were 1.4 million households with children under the age of 16 below the decency threshold, representing one in eight children. By the mid-1990s, the number had trebled to 4.2 million, representing one in three children (Goodman and Webb 1994). Underlying this trend is the increase in the poverty of lone parent households. In the mid-1990s, 7 per cent of UK households were lone parent households with children. Over 40 per cent were in the lowest income quintile and only 4 per cent were in the richest fifth of UK households. As a comparison and contrast, 22 per cent of UK households are male/female couple households without children: one in ten are in the lowest quintile and over one in three are in the highest income quintile (Goodman *et al.* 1997).

The trends in poverty and income inequality captured in Figure 4.9 are based on cross-sectional data. They tell us the proportion of people below the poverty line at particular points in time. However, longitudinal studies which track the culminative influence of disadvantage on health are highlighting the importance of people's (un)changing circumstances over time. Longitudinal studies of income dynamics are now underway in the UK and early findings indicate that most households 'hold their position' in the income distribution year by year. For example, a four-year study of income dynamics found that the majority of households never entered the poorest fifth of households, while the majority of poor households were on trajectories which kept them in poverty either continuously or with a short spell out of what was otherwise chronic poverty. Households with children were more likely to be persistently poor than other households (Jarvis and Jenkins 1997).

Most (65 per cent) of those in the poorest fifth of the income distribution are in receipt of means-tested benefits, with their income and living standards set by the social security system (Hills 1998). One in three people in Britain are in receipt of one or more of the major means-tested benefits, designed to provide a basic standard of living for those with inadequate incomes from other sources. Households on income support make up the largest group of benefit recipients and the largest group among Britain's poor (Department of Social Security (DSS) 1997). They therefore capture, simply but powerfully, the nature of contemporary poverty in the UK.

Parents and children make up the majority of those dependent on income support. There are 2.9 million children under the age of 16 – one in four of all children in Britain – living in households in receipt of income support together with 2 million parents (DSS 1997). The majority of the parents are women and most are caring for their children as lone mothers. Seventy per cent of households with children under 16 in receipt of income support are headed by a lone mother (DSS 1997).

The high level of welfare dependency among Britain's lone mothers is a recent trend. In 1971, around one in three (37 per cent) of lone mothers were receiving supplementary benefit, the precursor of income support (Burghes 1993). In 1999, the proportion is twice as high. Behind this trend lie changes in the composition of the lone parent population. An increasing proportion of lone mothers are younger and single (never married) lone mothers with younger children, for whom opportunities for well paid employment are often limited.

The increase in the number and proportion of families dependent on income support has occurred across a period in which its value has fallen relative to average disposable income. As a result, claimants have been getting relatively poorer, less able to afford what are regarded as necessities by the majority of the population (Bradshaw 1993). A series of studies have found that current levels of state benefits are insufficient to meet the basic needs of those who depend on them. While the evidence from longitudinal studies argues for extra protection for the living standards of expectant mothers and families, the income shortfall is particularly pronounced among households expecting and already caring for children (Bradshaw 1993; Oldfield and Yu 1993; Middleton *et al.* 1997). The structure of income support, with its combination of personal allowances and premiums, further disadvantages particular types of families. Again, the inequalities go against the grain of evidence from epidemiological research. It has been found that benefit rates are insufficient to meet the costs of an adequate diet for single expectant mothers and underestimate the costs of meeting the basic needs of younger children (especially those under 2 years of age) relative to older children (Dallison and Lobstein 1997; Middleton *et al.* 1997). The rates paid to one and two parent families also underestimate the relative cost of providing a basic standard of living for lone parent families (Berthoud and Ford 1996).

When income falls short of health needs, lifestyles are more likely to be designed around current threats to family survival than future risks to individual health (Graham 1998). As noted in the previous section, cutting back on food is the major strategy for making ends meet. As a result, diets have a limited nutrient base, with two or three foods providing the majority of nutrients (Dowler and Calvert 1995). While parents protect their children from the worse effects of nutritional deprivation, a significant proportion of women in claimant households have diets deficient in key nutrients (Lobstein 1991; Dowler and Calvert 1995). However, despite the pressure to economize, the prevalence of cigarette smoking in claimant households is high. Cigarette smoking can be experienced as a basic necessity in a lifestyle stripped of personal luxuries: as mothers have explained to researchers, a habit laid down in adolescence is hard to break in circumstances where past and current hardship is set to run on into the future (Graham 1989, 1993). A quantitative study of lone mothers has confirmed these qualitative insights. Dorsett and Marsh (1998) define mothers as living in 'severe hardship' if they were facing three or more hardships from a list which included having two or more problem debts and being unable to afford two or more basic foods. In an analysis which included the effects of other dimensions of low socio-economic status, living in severe hardship was found to be the primary deterrent to quitting smoking (Dorsett and Marsh 1998). Among the factors contributing to high levels of hardship among claimant families is their location on the wrong side of the process of polarization which has been reshaping Britain's class structure in the 1980s and 1990s.

Socio-economic polarization

The 1980s and 1990s have been marked out by a polarization in the socio-economic circumstances of households. Underlying this process have been changes in the structure of the labour market and in the relationships of employment which tie individuals to it, changes which have had a more negative effect on the manual and unskilled workforce than on non-manual and professional groups. The 1970s and 1980s saw

Figure 4.10 Households of working age with no member in paid work, UK 1979–97

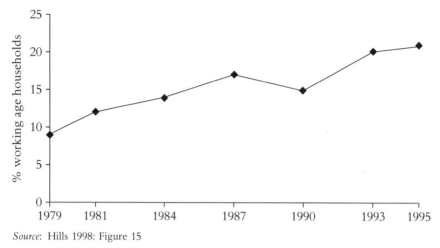

Source: Hills 1998: Figure 15

a major contraction of manual jobs in the UK, and unemployment rates for men in unskilled manual socio-economic groups rose from 15 per cent in the early 1970s to 30 per cent in the early 1990s. In contrast, the number of people in managerial and professional occupations increased sharply and recession and restructuring have had relatively little impact on employment rates of men in higher class groups. Men in social class I and II saw their rates of unemployment rise from 1 per cent to 5 per cent between the early 1970s and early 1990s (ONS 1998). Not only have opportunities for paid work become more unequal; so too have opportunities for high pay. Among adults in employment, the earnings of high paid workers have risen much faster than those in low paid jobs, widening earning differentials among both men and women (Hills 1998).

Changes in the structure of the labour market and in the dispersal of earnings have been associated with a more far-reaching change. They have fuelled a redistribution of employment between households. Across the 1980s and 1990s there has been a rapid shift away from households containing a mix of employed and non-employed adults and a corresponding increase in two-earner and no-earner households (Gregg and Wadsworth 1996). The proportion of no-earner households has doubled since the late 1970s, from less than one in ten households in 1979 to more than one in five in 1995 (Figure 4.10).

Changes in household composition, and in particular the growth in single parent and childless single adult households, explain some of the growth in no-earner households. To take account of this demographic

Figure 4.11 Employment in two-adult households, Britain 1975–93

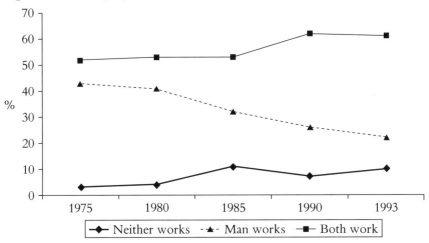

Source: Gregg and Wadsworth 1996: Table 8.1

trend, Figure 4.11 is restricted to the dominant household form. It focuses on two-adult households, which represent about 60 per cent of all households in Britain. As the figure indicates, male-earner households have given way to two-earner and no-earner households. In less than two decades, the proportion of two-adult households with a male breadwinner fell by half, from 43 per cent in 1975 to 22 per cent in 1993. Across this period, the proportion of no-earner households trebled, from 3 per cent to 10 per cent, and the proportion of two-earner households climbed from around 50 per cent to over 60 per cent. The upward trend in no-earner households reflects the toll of increasing unemployment. However, new jobs have disproportionately been taken by those living in households where another member is already in work (Gregg and Wadsworth 1996).

The changing household distribution of work has fuelled a wider process of socio-economic polarization. During the 1980s, the clumping of households on middle incomes began to break up. In its place, a new income distribution has emerged, characterized by high and rising real incomes for working households and low and stagnant incomes for non-working households (Jenkins 1996; Cowell *et al.* 1997; Hills 1998). For no-earner households dependent on means-tested benefits, real incomes have not even been stagnant. As noted in the previous section, they have declined.

The process of socio-economic polarization not only is evident in the patterns of household employment and income, but also is reflected, and reinforced, in the changing patterns of housing tenure. In the mid-1970s, households at all levels of income were found in social housing (in homes rented from local authorities and housing associations). Only in the richest fifth of households did the proportion in social housing drop below one-third (Hills 1997). The picture at the end of the 1990s is very different. Social housing is housing for the poor. Less than 5 per cent of the richest fifth of households live in this sector, while it provides homes for over 40 per cent of the poorest fifth of households. Not only is tenure stratified by income, but also it is stratified by employment status. In the owner-occupied sector, the majority of head of households (77 per cent) are in paid employment. In the social housing sector, the majority of household heads (63 per cent) are economically inactive (ONS 1998).

The process by which the socio-economic circumstances of house-holds are polarizing has a spatial dimension. Industrial decline in the UK has been concentrated in those regions and areas whose economies depended on manufacturing and mining (Champion and Townsend 1990). The early 1990s recession hit the service sector as much as the industrial sector, extending the spatial distribution of disadvantage to include the south of England as well as the traditionally disadvantaged areas of northern England, Wales and Scotland. The clustering of dis-advantage is captured in deprivation indices, based on measures of low socio-economic status such as unemployment, low skilled employment, tenure and car ownership. These indices reveal the area concentration of disadvantage, with the highest rates in inner city areas and peripheral housing estates (Green 1996; Sloggett and Joshi 1998).

The areas in which poor people live are also poor areas: they contain more health hazards and provide fewer health amenities than areas popu-lated by better-off households. With respect to hazards, traffic volume tends to be higher in disadvantaged urban areas, with a resulting increase both in the rates of road traffic accidents and in car vehicle emissions (British Medical Association (BMA) 1997; Quality of Urban Air Review Group (QUARG) 1998). Motor vehicles are the major cause of accidental death among children over the age of 5 and an important contributor to the socio-economic gradient in childhood mortality (Quick 1991). Emissions from vehicles are the major cause of air pollution and a con-tributory cause of respiratory disease (Committee on the Medical Effects of Air Pollution (COMEAP) 1998). While exposure to hazards goes with living in poorer areas, access to amenities is a feature of more advantaged areas. A study in the Scottish city of Glasgow compared two contrasting areas displaying low and high levels of aggregate deprivation (as measured by male unemployment, overcrowding, households without a car and households in social class IV/V). Despite the fact that residents in better-off areas were much more likely to have a car to access

Figure 4.12   Family characteristics of lone and couple families

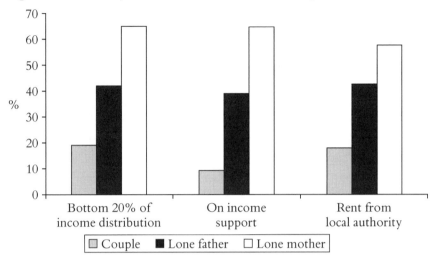

Source: Benzeval 1998b: Table 7

health-promoting resources outside their local area, local levels of provision were consistently higher in better-off areas. This was true with
respect to shops, recreational facilities, public transport and primary
health care services (Macintyre 1997).

   As the trends in employment, household income, housing tenure and
area amenities indicate, dimensions of socio-economic disadvantage are
both clustering and polarizing in the UK. Those most vulnerable to
poor health and premature mortality find themselves on the wrong side
of this process of polarization: living in households in which there is no
one in employment, in social housing and in neighbourhoods high
in health risks and low in health resources. These groups represent a
mixture of the traditionally poor, like male unskilled manual workers
and their families, whose lives have traditionally been punctured by unemployment and framed by low income. The process of polarization
is linked, too, to newer social divisions, built around housing tenure,
welfare dependency and lone motherhood. A recent analysis of the
socio-economic circumstances of lone mothers, lone fathers and (heterosexual) couple parents illustrates the extent to which these dimensions
of disadvantage overlap (Benzeval 1998b). While the majority of lone
mothers were in the lowest income quintile, not in full-time employment, on income support and in social housing, only a minority of couple
parents were in these disadvantaged categories (Figure 4.12). While the

majority of lone mothers were under 35 years, the majority of mothers (and fathers) in couple households were over 35. Evidence from longitudinal studies points to the socio-economic patterning of lone motherhood, with girls born to fathers in manual occupations more likely to take on the risks and rewards of lone motherhood in their adult lives (Figure 4.8).

The polarizing of lifecourse patterns – and with them living standards and life chances – has profound implications for the socio-economic gradients in men's and women's health. At the least, it means that the class structure no longer consists of a hierarchy of unequal but relatively stable positions. Increasingly, it is a structure composed of unequal and divergent socio-economic trajectories.

Conclusion

This chapter has turned the spotlight on socio-economic inequalities in men's and women's health in the UK. It is a spotlight which means that the influence of other structures of inequality have been obscured. It is important to remember that the analysis it offers is both partial and preliminary. It is not only an individual's social class and gender which have health effects: an individual's health takes the strain – physical and psychological – of all the structures of inequality to which the person is exposed.

The chapter began by noting that, while there are important differences in the socio-economic gradients in men's and women's health, the dominant pattern is one in which class privilege brings health advantage. Whether male or female, our class background and our class trajectory is written into how well and how long we live.

The central sections of the chapter reviewed research from social epidemiology and social policy which explores the links between class inequality and health inequality among men and women. It noted that research has focused on individual level links, where class inequality takes its shape in health related behaviours and in the material and psychosocial environments in which they are sustained. Further, research exploring how socio-economic status patterns an individual's exposure to behavioural, material and psychosocial risks has only recently engaged with gender. There is still a lot to learn about how gender structures and mediates these exposures. There is much to learn, too, about how processes beyond the behaviour and environment of the individual work their way through into people's expectations and experiences of health. Yet it is these structural factors – operating at the area, national and supranational level – which play a key role in determining the distribution of life chances and living standards, both between socio-economic groups and between men and women. It is changes in these macro-level systems, too, which are fuelling changes in the distribution of life chances and living standards.

The final section of the chapter focused on these broader trends. It described how, in the UK, socio-economic changes are widening inequalities in the opportunity to move into and along the lifecourse trajectories associated with better health and longer life. While research is only beginning to map the lifecourse patterns, it suggests that men born into higher socio-economic groups can expect to occupy advantaged positions with respect to employment, income and housing tenure in their adult life. Their advantaged positions in the labour and housing markets increase their command over the material, psychosocial and behavioural resources associated with good health. For women in higher socio-economic groups, their household circumstances – whether they are married without children or a lone mother with them – are likely to structure their access to these protected and privileged lifecourse trajectories. In contrast, men and women born into lower socio-economic groups face the prospect of downward socio-economic trajectories. These pathways into and through adulthood are marked out by low and declining living standards, sustained on means-tested benefits and in social housing in poor neighbourhoods. These pathways offer few opportunities to escape health damaging material and psychosocial environments and to break health damaging patterns of behaviour.

In the UK, this process of polarization occurred across two decades in which inequality was off the political agenda. From 1979 to 1997, Britain was led by a Conservative government which recognized that there were individual differences in health and wealth, but rejected explanations that these differences reflected socially structured inequalities. The result was a free market approach to economic, social and fiscal policy in which inequalities resulting from labour market restructuring and the emergence of new patterns of family life were magnified rather than moderated.

As the example of the UK suggests, and comparative research confirms, national state policies play an important part in filtering the effects of social and socio-economic change. Change – whether at the level of the transnational corporation and the global labour market or in our patterns of cohabitation and parenthood – is not inevitably linked to widening inequalities in health and opportunity. Whether and how far social and economic change results in widening inequalities depends on national state policies: social, economic and fiscal (Bradshaw 1996; Breen and Rottman 1998). The New Labour government, elected in 1997, has launched a public health strategy built around the twin aims of improving the UK's health and reducing health inequalities. It is a strategy built on the recognition that 'tackling inequalities in general is the best way of tackling health inequalities in particular' (Secretary of State for Health 1998). The detail of the government's strategy has still to emerge and take effect. Nonetheless, the renewed political commitment to reducing the socio-economic gradient in health suggests that the UK still remains an instructive case study through which to track the links between inequality and the lives, and deaths, of men and women.

Acknowledgements

I would like to thank Stephen Stansfeld for unpublished data from the Whitehall II Study and Tanya Richardson for moral support and help with typing the chapter.

References

Barker, D. (1998) *Mothers, Babies and Health in Later Life*. London: Churchill Livingstone.

Benzeval, M. (1998a) Poverty and health, *Health Variations*, 1: 12–13.

Benzeval, M. (1998b) The self-reported health status of lone parents, *Social Science and Medicine*, 46(10): 1337–53.

Berthoud, R. and Ford, R. (1996) *Relative Needs: Variations in the Living Standards of Different Types of Household*. London: Policy Studies Institute.

Bradshaw, J. (1993) *Household Budgets and Living Standards*. York: Joseph Rowntree Foundation.

Bradshaw, J. (1996) *The Employment of Lone Parents: A Comparison of Policy in 20 Countries*. London: Family Policy Studies Centre.

Breen, R. and Rottman, R. (1998) Is the national state the appropriate geographical unit for class analysis?, *Sociology*, 32(1): 1–21.

British Medical Association (BMA) (1997) *Road Transport and Health*. London: BMA.

Brown, G. and Harris, T. (1978) *The Social Origins of Depression*. London: Tavistock.

Burghes, L. (1993) *One Parent Families: Policy Options for the 1990s*. York: Family Policy Studies Centre.

Burrows, R. and Nettleton, S. (1997) British women's smoking in the employers and managers socio-economic group, *Health Promotion International*, 12(3): 209–14.

Burstrom, B., Diderichsen, F., Shouls, S. and Whitehead, M. (in press) Lone mothers in Sweden: trends in health and socio-economic circumstances, 1979–1995, in *Journal of Epidemiology and Community Health*.

Champion, A. and Townsend, A. (1990) *Contemporary Britain: A Geographical Perspective*. London: Edward Arnold.

Colhoun, H. and Prescott-Clarke, P. (eds) (1996) *Health Survey for England 1994*. London: HMSO.

Committee on the Medical Effects of Air Pollution (COMEAP) (1998) *Quantification of the Effects of Air Pollution on Health in the United Kingdom*. London: Stationery Office.

Corti, L. and Dex, S. (1995) Informal carers and employment, *Employment Gazette*, 103: 101–7.

Cowell, F. A., Jenkins, S. P. and Litchfield, J. A. (1997) The changing shape of the UK income distribution: kernel density estimates, in J. Hills (ed.) *New Inequalities: The Changing Distribution of Income and Wealth in the United Kingdom*. Cambridge: Cambridge University Press.

Dallison, J. and Lobstein, T. (1997) *Poor Expectations: Poverty and Undernourishment in Pregnancy*. London: NCH (National Children's Home) Action for Children and the Maternity Alliance.

Davey Smith, G., Blane, D. and Bartley, M. (1994) Explanations for socio-economic differentials in mortality, *European Journal of Public Health*, 4: 131–44.

Davey Smith, G., Hart, C., Blane, D., Gillis, C. and Hawthorne, V. (1997) Lifetime socio-economic position and mortality: prospective observational study, *British Medical Journal*, 314: 547–52.

Davey Smith, G., Hart, C., Hole, D. *et al.* (1998) Education and occupational social class: which is the more important indicator of mortality risk?, *Journal of Epidemiology and Community Health*, 52: 153–60.

Dennehy, A. (1998) Keeping mum: the condition of working class women in late 20th century England. Unpublished doctoral thesis, University of Bristol.

Department of Social Security (DSS) (1997) *Social Security Statistics 1997*. London: Stationery Office.

Dorsett, R. and Marsh, A. (1998) *The Health Trap: Poverty, Smoking and Lone Parenthood*. London: Policy Studies Institute.

Dowler, E. and Calvert, C. (1995) *Nutrition and Diet in Lone Parent Families in London*. London: Family Policy Studies Centre.

Drever, F. and Bunting, J. (1997) Patterns and trends in male mortality, in F. Drever and M. Whitehead (eds) *Health Inequalities*, series DS no. 15. London: Stationery Office.

Elliot, J. and Huppert, F. (1991) In sickness and in health: associations between physical and mental wellbeing, employment and parental status in a nationwide sample of married women, *Psychological Medicine*, 21: 515–24.

Emslie, C., Hunt, K. and Macintyre, S. (1999a) Problematising gender, work and health: the relationship between gender, occupational grade, working conditions and minor morbidity in full-time bank employees, *Social Science and Medicine*, 48(1): 33–48.

Emslie, C., Hunt, K. and Macintyre, S. (1999b) Gender differences in minor morbidity amongst full-time employees of a British University, *Journal of Epidemiology and Community Health*, 53(8): 465–75.

Filakti, H. and Fox, J. (1995) Differences in mortality by housing tenure and by car access from the OPCS Longitudinal Study, *Population Trends*, 81: 27–30.

Giddens, A. (1991) *Modernity and Self-Identity*. London: Polity Press.

Goodman, A. and Webb, S. (1994) *For Richer, For Poorer: The Changing Distribution of Income in the United Kingdom*. London: Institute of Fiscal Studies.

Goodman, A., Johnson, P. and Webb, S. (1997) *Inequality in the UK*. Oxford: Oxford University Press.

Graham, H. (1989) Women and smoking in the United Kingdom: the implications for health promotion, *Health Promotion International*, 3(4): 371–82.

Graham, H. (1993) *When Life's a Drag: Women, Smoking and Disadvantage*. London: HMSO.

Graham, H. (1998) Health at risk: poverty and national health strategies, in L. Doyal (ed.) *Women and Health Services*. Buckingham: Open University Press.

Graham, H. and Hunt, S. (1994) Women's smoking and measures of women's socio-economic status in the United Kingdom, *Health Promotion International*, 9: 81–8.

Green, A. (1996) Aspects of the changing geography of poverty and wealth, in J. Hills (ed.) *New Inequalities: The Changing Distribution of Income and Wealth in the United Kingdom*. Cambridge: Cambridge University Press.

Gregg, P. and Wadsworth, J. (1996) More work in fewer households, in J. Hills (ed.) *New Inequalities: The Changing Distribution of Income and Wealth in the United Kingdom*. Cambridge: Cambridge University Press.

Harding, S., Bethune, A., Maxwell, R. and Brown, J. (1997) Mortality trends using the Longitudinal Study, in F. Drever and M. Whitehead (eds) *Health Inequalities*, series DS no. 15. London: Stationery Office.

Haskey, J. (1998) One parent families and their dependent children in Great Britain, *Population Trends*, 91: 5–13.

Hills, J. (1997) *The Future of Welfare: A Guide to the Debate*. York: Joseph Rowntree Foundation.

Hills, J. (1998) *Income and Wealth: The Latest Evidence*. York: Joseph Rowntree Foundation.

Hunt, K. and Macintyre, S. (in press) Sexe et inégalités sociales en santé, in H. Grandjean (ed.) *Inégalités et disparités sociales en santé*. Paris: La Découverte.

Jarvis, S. and Jenkins, S. P. (1997) Low income dynamics in 1990s Britain, *Fiscal Studies*, 18(2): 123–42.

Jenkins, S. (1996) Recent trends in the UK income distribution: what happened and why?, *Oxford Review of Economic Policy*, 12(1): 29–45.

Johansson, S. R. (1991) Welfare, mortality and gender: continuity and change in explanations for male/female mortality differences over three generations, *Continuity and Change*, 6: 135–78.

Kempson, E., Bryson, A. and Rawlingson, K. (1994) *Hard Times? How Poor Families Make Ends Meet*. London: Policy Studies Institute.

Kiernan, K. (1989) The family: formation and fission, in H. Joshi (ed.) *The Changing Population of Britain*. Oxford: Blackwell.

Kuh, D. and Ben-Shlomo, Y. (eds) (1997) *A Lifecourse Approach to Chronic Disease Epidemiology*. Oxford: Oxford Medical.

Lantz, P. M., House, J. S., Lepkauski, J. M., Williams, D. R., Mero, R. P. and Chen, J. (1998) Socio-economic factors, health behaviours and mortality, *Journal of the American Medical Association*, 279(21): 1703–8.

Lobstein, T. (1991) *The Nutrition of Women on Low Income*. London: London Food Commission.

Lundberg, O. (1991) The impact of childhood living conditions on illness and mortality in adulthood, *Social Science and Medicine*, 36(8): 1047–52.

Macintyre, S. (1997) What are spatial effects and how can we measure them?, in A. Dale (ed.) *Exploiting National Survey and Census Data: The Role of Locality and Spatial Effects*, Catherine Marsh Centre for Census and Survey Research occasional paper 12. Manchester: University of Manchester.

Macintyre, S. and Hunt, K. (1997) Socio-economic position, gender and health: how do they interact?, *Journal of Health Psychology*, 2(3): 315–34.

Macran, S., Clark, L. and Joshi, H. (1996) Women's health: dimensions and differentials, *Social Science and Medicine*, 42(9): 1203–16.

Marmot, M. G. and Davey Smith, G. (1997) Socio-economic differentials in health, *Journal of Health Psychology*, 2(3): 283–96.

Marmot, M. G., Shipley, M. J. and Rose, G. (1984) Inequalities in death: specific explanations of a general pattern, *Lancet*, (1): 1003–6.

Marmot, M. G., Bosma, H., Hemingway, H., Brunner, E. and Stansfeld, S. (1997) Contribution of job control and other risk factors to social variations in coronary heart disease incidence, *Lancet*, 350: 235–39.

Mheen, D. van de (1998) *Inequalities in Health: To be Continued? A Lifecourse Perspective on Socio-economic Inequalities in Health*. Rotterdam: Erasmus University.

Middleton, S., Ashworth, K. and Braithwaite, I. (1997) *Small Fortunes: Spending on Children, Childhood Poverty and Parental Sacrifice*. York: Joseph Rowntree Foundation.

Nazroo, J. (1997) *The Health of Britain's Ethnic Minorities: Findings from a National Survey*. London: Policy Studies Institute.

Office for National Statistics (ONS) (1998) *Living in Britain: Results from the 1996 General Household Survey*. London: Stationery Office.

Oldfield, N. and Yu, A. C. S. (1993) *The Cost of a Child: Living Standards for the 1990s*. London: Child Poverty Action Group.

Phillips, A. N. and Davey Smith, G. (1991) How independent are 'independent' effects? Relative risk estimation when correlated exposures are measured imprecisely, *Journal of Clinical Epidemiology*, 44: 1223–31.

Popay, J., Bartley, M. and Owen, C. (1993) Gender inequalities in health: social position, affective disorders and minor physical morbidity, *Social Science and Medicine*, 36(1): 21–32.

Power, C. (1991) Social and economic background and class inequalities in health among adults, *Social Science and Medicine*, 32(4): 411–17.

Power, C. and Matthews, S. (1997) Origins of health inequalities in a national population sample, *Lancet*, 350: 1584–5.

Power, C., Manor, O. and Fox, A. J. (1991) *Health and Class: The Early Years*. London: Chapman Hall.

Power, C., Matthews, S. and Manor, O. (1996) Inequalities in self-rated health in the 1958 birth cohort: life time social circumstances or social mobility?, *British Medical Journal*, 313: 449–53.

Prescott-Clarke, P. and Primatesta, P. (eds) (1998) *Health Survey for England 1996*. London: Stationery Office.

Quality of Urban Air Review Group (QUARG) (1998) *Urban Air Quality in the United Kingdom*. London: Department of Environment, Transport and the Regions.

Quick, A. (1991) *Unequal Risks*. London: Socialist Health Association.

Rose, D. and O'Reilly, K. (1997) *Constructing Classes: Towards a New Classification for the UK*. Swindon: Office for National Statistics/Economic and Social Research Council.

Secretary of State for Health (1998) *Our Healthier Nation: A Contract for Health*. London: Stationery Office.

Skeggs, B. (1997) *Formations of Class and Gender*. London: Sage.

Sloggett, A. and Joshi, H. (1998) Indicators of deprivation in people and places: longitudinal perspectives, *Environment and Planning*, A30: 1055–76.

Smith, J. and Harding, S. (1997) Mortality of women and men using alternative social classifications, in F. Drever and M. Whitehead (eds) *Health Inequalities*, series DS no. 15. London: Stationery Office.

Stronks, K. (1997) *Socio-economic Inequalities in Health: Individual Choice or Social Circumstances*. Rotterdam: Erasmus University.

Stronks, K., van de Mheen, H. and Mackenbach, J. P. (1998) A higher prevalence of health problems in low income groups: does it reflect relative deprivation?, *Journal of Epidemiology and Community Health*, 52: 548–57.

Weich, S. and Lewis, G. (1998) Material standard of living, social class and the prevalence of the common mental disorders, *Journal of Epidemiology and Community Health*, 52: 8–14.

Whelan, C. (1993) The role of social support in mediating the psychological consequences of economic stress, *Sociology of Health and Illness*, 15(1): 86–101.

Whitehead, M. (1997) Life and death across the millennium, in F. Drever and M. Whitehead (eds) *Health Inequalities*, series DS no. 15. London: Stationery Office.

Woods, R. and Williams, N. (1995) Must the gap widen before it can be narrowed? Long term trends in social class mortality differentials, *Continuity and Change*, 10(1): 105–37.

five

Gender and inequalities in health across the lifecourse

Sara Arber and Helen Cooper

Introduction

This chapter examines gender differences in the nature of inequalities in health at three stages of the lifecourse – childhood, working life and later life. Gender roles and responsibilities are socially constructed in ways which vary across the lifecourse. Similarly, ageing and old age as categories are culturally produced and socially structured, varying over time and between societies (Arber and Ginn 1995).

During the twentieth century there have been radical changes in actual and expected gender roles, as well as in norms as to age-related behaviour, especially young people's sexuality and participation in education. Societal expectations about the roles and behaviour of older people have been more stable, although some writers (Evandrou 1997) argue that when the cohort of 'baby boomers' enter later life in the early years of the twenty-first century, this will herald new ideas about the appropriate behaviour of older men and women. Thus, age and gender differences in health are likely to reflect the socially constructed nature of gender roles and expectations regarding chronological age. We may therefore expect the nature of inequalities in health for men and women to vary for different age groups.

In this chapter, we use British data to examine inequalities in health among men and among women at three different stages of the lifecourse in order to question whether the patterns of inequalities differ by gender, and to illustrate our contention that different factors should be considered at different stages of the lifecourse. Our analyses are not just confined to social class inequalities. In childhood, we also consider inequalities by the child's family structure, parental employment status and housing tenure. For men and women of working age, we examine inequalities by family structure, education, social class, employment status, and material circumstances (as indicated by car ownership and housing tenure). In older adults, we consider inequalities by occupational class, marital status, household income and housing tenure.

Generations and the lifecourse

The health and other characteristics of women and men are influenced by their prior lifecourse (Wadsworth 1997). This is most vividly seen in later life, since the financial circumstances of older adults are intimately tied to their previous role in the labour market and thus their pension acquisition (Ginn and Arber 1996, 1998). For women in mid-life, their health and well-being is influenced by their history of childbearing and their role as parents. Increasingly, health during working life is structured according to position in the labour market, which itself is closely linked to earlier success in the educational sphere (Lahelma and Rahkonen 1997). Thus, a lifecourse approach 'provides a framework for analysing the various influences which contribute to the life experience of different groups of individuals at particular stages of their lives. A life course approach emphasizes the interlinkage between phases of the life course, rather than seeing each phase in isolation' (Arber and Evandrou 1993: 9). It takes social change seriously and sees lives as dynamic and responsive to changed circumstances and opportunities, but often in gendered ways.

Some writers have considered the variations in attitudes and behaviour among birth cohorts, or whole generations. Mannheim (1952) linked the process of the formation of generations to social change, arguing not only that generations relate to being born in the same era, but also that those who live through a period of rapid social change develop a separate 'historical-social conscience' or collective identity, which influences their attitudes and behaviour and distinguishes them from preceeding and succeeding generations. Such 'historical or social generations' are distinguished by the historical experiences they have shared, which in turn have shaped their common vision of the world.

In terms of attitudes towards gender roles, the 1960s in Britain marked a major change, reflected in legislation such as the Abortion Act 1967 and the Equal Pay Act 1970. We would expect the effects of such social changes to be greatest for those in their formative years at that time, especially women. Gender is a fundamental dimension throughout the lifecourse, distinguishing between men and women as to what is considered appropriate behaviour in any cultural context; but this will vary for different birth cohorts or historical/social generations.

Other writers have focused on broad age groups, as for example, in Laslett's (1989) division of the lifecourse into 'four ages'. His First Age is conceptualized as the increasingly extended period of education; the Second Age corresponds to working life, and his Third Age is conceptualized as one of opportunity following retirement from paid employment and after childrearing. He also distinguishes a 'Fourth Age', as one of 'decline and decrepitude' at the end of life.

Gender inequalities within one life stage may influence and be predicated on gender inequalities in another. For example, the extent to which women forgo paid employment to raise children will lead to financial penalties both during their working life and in retirement because of lower private pension contributions (Ginn and Arber 1996, 1998, 1999a), but the extent of these penalties is likely to vary by social class and according to the woman's marital relationship, with lone mothers suffering the greatest financial penalties of parenthood.

Inequalities in health among men and women in Britain

Aims and methods

Our discussion of the nature of inequalities in health among women and men will examine three broad life stages: childhood, working age and the retirement years or later life. A tripartite division of the lifecourse based on chronological age is crude, since ideally the analysis should be subdivided according to participation in the labour market, but it will allow an illustration of how different factors may be responsible for inequalities in women's and men's health at different phases of the lifecourse.

For each stage of the lifecourse, we present secondary analysis of nationally representative data from the British General Household Survey (GHS) for the 1990s. The GHS conducts interviews with all adults living in about 10,000 households per year and achieved a response rate of 80 per cent in 1994/5 (Bennett *et al.* 1996). As the GHS is a cross-sectional survey, it is not always possible to disentangle the direction of causation between some variables and ill health (for example, whether unemployment causes ill health or sickness leads to unemployment). Longitudinal studies, such as the British birth cohort studies (Fogelman 1983; Power *et al.* 1993) are of particular value in this respect, but there are no large British nationally representative longitudinal surveys which focus on mid-life or later life. A benefit of using the GHS for the present analysis is that comparable data are available for each stage of the lifecourse and the same questions are asked each year. The large sample size, especially when three years of GHS data are combined, makes it possible to reliably analyse small population subgroups, such as lone parents.

For children, limiting longstanding illness (LLI) is used as the measure of health, while for working age and older adults self-assessed health is used. For children under 16 years, the person assuming most responsibility for the child, usually the mother, is asked: 'Do(es) your child(ren) have any longstanding illness, disability or infirmity?' If the answer is 'Yes', the question continues 'Does this illness/disability limit your child's activities in any way?' Our analysis examines those who report that their child has a limiting longstanding illness (LLI). Self-assessed health is asked of adults and older people, but not children. It is measured by the GHS question: 'Over the last twelve months, would you say that your health has on the whole been good, fairly good or not good?' Poor self-assessed health has been shown to be a good predictor of mortality in other studies (Mossey and Shapiro 1982; Idler and Benyamini 1997).

Childhood

Social class has been a dominant concept in British research on inequalities in health among children, showing strong differentials in mortality and morbidity. The Black Report (Townsend and Davidson 1982) had a major influence on subsequent research (e.g. Fogelman 1983; Drever and Whitehead 1997; Acheson Report 1998), which has focused on analysing children's health by the social class of the head of household. However, research in Scotland has found weaker class gradients for adolescents (West 1988, 1997; West *et al.* 1990). West (1997) argues that the relative health equality in adolescence results from influences associated with school, peer group and youth culture, which cut across traditional class boundaries. Sweeting and West (1995) found that although family structure, especially living in a lone parent family, was associated with material deprivation, there was no association between deprivation at home and health status among adolescents.

Since the early 1970s there have been major changes in family structure in Britain. For example, a threefold increase in the number of lone parent families, with one-fifth living in a one parent family by 1996 (Church 1997), the majority of whom rely on state benefits (Dale 1995). Over the same period, there have been major structural changes in the labour market, particularly fluctuating levels of unemployment, and increased employment participation of mothers (Brannen *et al.* 1994; Glover and Arber 1995; Church 1997). These societal changes have led to a greater diversity of children's experiences and lifestyles depending on whether they are growing up in a no-earner family, a family where

Figure 5.1 Percentage reporting limiting longstanding illness (LLI) by socio-economic group of family unit head: girls and boys aged 0–15 years

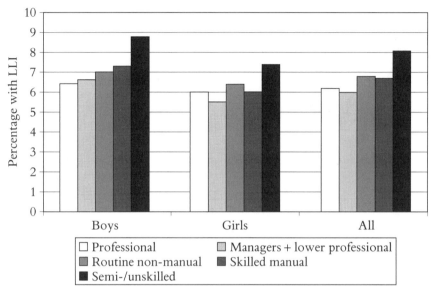

p (ns) for girls and boys; p < 0.05 for all children
Source: General Household Survey 1992/3, 1993/4 and 1994/5

the mother is a full-time housewife, or a dual-earner family. There may be a growing polarization of children's life chances according to the work status of their parents and their family structure, which supersede occupational social class as a dimension of stratification and health inequality. However, research still focuses on occupational social class as the primary determinant of health inequalities among children (Drever and Whitehead 1997; Acheson Report 1998).

We examine gender differences in inequalities in reported limiting longstanding illness among children from birth to 15 who live with one or both of their parents, using three years of General Household Survey data (1992–4) – in total over 15,000 boys and girls. A more detailed analysis is provided in Cooper *et al.* (1998). Social class is measured by the current or last occupation of the family unit head. Somewhat more boys than girls under 16 are reported to have a limiting longstanding illness, 7.6 per cent of boys and 6.3 per cent of girls.

Among British children aged under 16 in the early 1990s, there is only a small social class gradient in the percentage reporting LLI for both girls and boys and this variation is not statistically significant (see Figure 5.1). The percentages with LLI vary from 6.4 per cent among

Figure 5.2   Percentage reporting limiting longstanding illness (LLI) by family work status: girls and boys aged 0–15 years

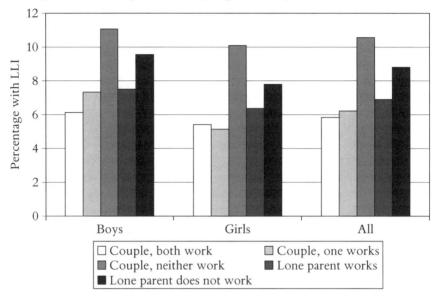

p < 0.001 for boys and girls
Source: General Household Survey 1992/3, 1993/4 and 1994/5

boys where the family head is in a professional or higher managerial occupation, to 8.8 per cent who come from a semi-skilled or unskilled class background. For girls there is a somewhat weaker and more in-consistent class gradient of reported limiting longstanding illness.

The child's family structure and the employment status of the parents has a greater influence on levels of chronic illness (Figure 5.2) than the social class of the family head. We distinguish children living with a couple (one or both of whom may be their natural parents), from children living with a lone parent, and distinguish these two types of family structures according to the employment status of the parent(s) to create a measure of 'family work status'. The lowest levels of LLI are reported among children living with a couple where both 'parents' are in paid employment (6 per cent of boys and 5.4 per cent of girls) and the highest LLI occurs for children where neither parent is employed (11 per cent of boys and 10 per cent of girls). LLI is also more commonly reported among children who live with a lone parent who is not working, but when a lone parent is employed the proportion reporting LLI is comparable to children in couples where at least one is earning.

However, the interpretation of these findings may be uncertain because of the possibility of reverse causation. For example, having a child with a chronic illness may restrict a lone parent's employment, but this is unlikely to account for the very high levels of chronic illness among children who live with a couple where neither is employed.

Children living in rented accommodation, which is mainly local authority (public) housing, have a higher level of chronic illness than those whose parents own their home, but the association reaches statistical significance only for girls. More girls living in rented accommodation are reported as having LLI (7 per cent), compared with 5 per cent living in owner-occupied housing. The comparable figures for boys are 8.2 per cent and 6.1 per cent.

Our analysis so far has explored patterns of children's health separately by social class, family structure and housing tenure; however, these three structural variables are themselves intercorrelated. For example, unemployment is much higher among those previously in lower social class occupations (Bartley and Owen 1996; Arber 1997) and lone parents are more likely to live in local authority housing than children who live with two parents (Cooper *et al.* 1998). In order to assess the relative importance of each of these structural variables, we conduct multivariate analysis separately for boys and girls. This enables us to examine the independent effects of each variable on reported LLI after controlling for the other variables and to compare the results for boys and girls. Logistic regression is used, since the dependent variable, whether or not the child has a limiting longstanding illness, is dichotomous. Age in paired years is included in all models.

Model A in Table 5.1 presents odds ratios of the likelihood of reporting LLI in each social class, compared with the reference category of children whose family head is currently in (or for those not in paid work, was last in) a professional or higher managerial occupation (which is set to 1.00). Children from semi- and unskilled families have higher odds ratios of LLI, but these differences reach statistical significance only for boys, who have a nearly 50 per cent higher odds of LLI than the reference category. These analyses suggest that social class, based on the current or last occupation of the family unit head, has only a limited influence on the likelihood of children having a chronic illness in Britain in the 1990s.

The child's family work status and housing tenure, as well as their social class and age, are included in Model B, Table 5.1. The child's family work status has a strong and significant effect on the likelihood of the child having a chronic illness, with a similar pattern found for girls and boys. Differences in health are more clearly related to the work status of their parents than to their family structure. Children

Table 5.1   Odds ratios of limiting longstanding illness (LLI), for boys and girls aged 0–15 years[1]

	Boys		*Girls*	
	Model A	*Model B*	*Model A*	*Model B*
Social class of family unit head	+	ns	ns	ns
Higher professional/managerial	1.00	1.00	1.00	1.00
Lower professional/managerial	1.03	0.98	0.89	0.81
Clerical, routine non-manual	1.16	0.95	1.13	0.90
Skilled manual	1.18	1.04	1.02	0.81
Semi-/unskilled manual	1.48★★	1.08	1.29	0.86
Family work status		++		+++
Couple, both work		1.00		1.00
Couple, one works		1.27★		1.08
Couple, neither work		1.72★★★		1.95★★★
Lone parent works		1.14		1.01
Lone parent does not work		1.65★★		1.45★
Housing		ns		+
Owner-occupier		1.00		1.00
Rented/local authority housing		1.20		1.36★
N	7,665		7,371	

Notes: [1] All models control for age in paired years
  ★ Significance of difference from the reference category: ★ $p < 0.05$; ★★ $p < 0.01$; ★★★ $p < 0.001$
  + Significance of variable in the model: + $p < 0.05$; ++ $p < 0.01$; +++ $p < 0.001$
Source: General Household Survey 1992/3, 1993/4, 1994/5

living with a couple where neither 'parent' is employed have nearly twice the odds of LLI compared with children whose parents are both employed. Children with an employed lone parent have comparable rates of chronic illness to children with two working parents, but for children whose lone parent is not employed, the odds ratio of LLI is increased by 65 per cent for boys and 45 per cent for girls. As mentioned above, there is the possibility of reverse causation where the parent's ability to engage in paid employment is restricted by having a sick child. Children living in privately rented or local authority housing also have elevated odds of LLI, after including class and family work status in the model, but this reaches statistical significance only for girls.

Once family work status and housing tenure are included in Model B, the association of chronic illness with the family's social class is no longer significant for boys. There is no indication of any higher levels of LLI among children in semi-skilled and unskilled families, which suggests a concentration of non-employment among lower class families, who are also more likely to live in local authority housing. Thus, our results show that measures of family structure, parental work status and housing tenure are more closely associated than social class with levels of reported chronic illness for children under 16. However, variations in children's health cannot be attributed to family structure *per se*, since the health of both boys and girls living in couple and lone parent families is adversely affected by their parent's non-employment. We conclude that in the 1990s, parental employment is paramount in influencing a child's health status, irrespective of the gender of the child.

This section has shown that the patterns of health inequalities are similar for boys and girls, but that the traditional basis of inequality according to occupational social class of family head has given way in the 1990s to other factors, especially the employment status of their parents, which is more closely tied to material deprivation than the traditional measure of father's social class. Our findings are likely to reflect major historical generational changes. For example, children under 16 in Britain in the 1990s were born after 1979, a time when unemployment increased and the Conservative government introduced sweeping reforms to the welfare state which increased owner-occupation leading to a residualization of local authority housing, and increased income inequality (Wilkinson 1996). In addition, this period saw an increase in the proportion of lone parent families, resulting mainly from higher divorce rates (Church 1997).

This contrasts with earlier studies of inequalities in health in the 1970s and 1980s (Townsend and Davidson 1982; Fogelman 1983) which focused on cohorts of children born in the late 1950s and 1960s, a time of relative prosperity, low levels of unemployment and reductions in income disparities. For this generation of children, class based on the position of their father in the labour market provided the most salient indicator of material disadvantage. Whereas, in the 1990s, the key material divide for children seems to be whether their parent is in paid employment or not, rather than their parent's class position within the occupational structure. Our analysis of children shows that the factors influencing health inequalities are similar for boys and girls.

The working ages

Analysis of gender differences in health inequalities during the main years of working life, defined here as 20–59, is complex, because of the need to take into account how women's (and men's) family roles, as well as their socio-economic position, impact on health. Until the early 1990s, most inequalities research on this stage of the lifecourse focused on occupational class inequalities in men's mortality and morbidity, with less attention paid to inequalities in health among British women (Townsend and Davidson 1982; Drever and Whitehead 1997; Acheson 1998). It is also important to go beyond a social class framework and consider how employment status and educational qualifications are associated with social variations in health (Arber 1997).

An ongoing debate in Britain has been whether a woman's class should be measured by her own occupation irrespective of her marital status – 'the individualistic' approach, or her husband's occupation if she is married, and her own occupation if she is not – the 'conventional' approach (Goldthorpe 1983; Arber 1997). The latter is still used in British government publications (e.g. Bennett *et al.* 1996; Drever and Whitehead 1997) and most other research. Arber (1989, 1997) has discussed the problems of using the 'conventional' approach, arguing that for married people, it is advantageous to use the occupational class, employment status and educational qualifications of both partners when analysing women's *and* men's health. However, where indicators relating to just one partner must be used, the individualistic approach may in future be more appropriate since it has the advantage of conceptual clarity, as well as capturing the recent growth in women's employment (Brannen *et al.* 1994; Hakim 1996), and the greater fluidity in marital status (Kiernan and Estaugh 1993; Buck *et al.* 1994).

Since the late 1980s, research has examined whether structural factors, such as social class and material disadvantage, are associated in a similar way with inequalities in women's and men's health (Arber 1989, 1991; Bartley *et al.* 1992; Macran *et al.* 1994, 1996; Arber 1997; Lahelma and Rahkonen 1997). These researchers have stressed the importance of analysing women's health, in terms of both their structural position within society and their family roles. However, less attention has been devoted to how men's health is related to their family roles.

Early work on marital and parental status and women's health was cast in a role analytic framework, examining to what extent additional roles, such as the parental role and paid employment, had beneficial or adverse consequences for women's health (e.g. Nathanson 1980; Verbrugge 1983; Arber *et al.* 1985). Research on marital status and health (e.g. Verbrugge 1979; Morgan 1980; Anson 1989; Wyke and Ford 1992) has consistently shown that divorced and separated people have poorer health than married people, and that single men, but not single women, report poorer health than those who are married. Despite the growth in cohabitation since the late 1970s (Kiernan and Estaugh 1993), we know less about its association with health. Similarly, there has been a neglect of research on parental roles and health, especially in relation to lone parenthood (although Popay and Jones (1990) is a notable exception). A major change since the late 1970s has been the growth in the proportion of women bringing up children as lone parents (Church 1997). This represents a key gender difference, since few men bring up children as lone fathers.

It is essential to examine how socio-economic circumstances, together with marital and parental roles, influence inequalities in health, and to assess whether the nature of these inequalities in health are gendered. A model of the types of variables influencing health during the working ages was discussed in Arber (1997). The key structural variables which influence an individual's health are related to their labour market position, that is, occupational class and employment status, both of which are influenced by the individual's level of educational qualifications. Family roles are likely to influence health. However, whether a woman becomes a lone parent and her age at childbearing may also be influenced by her class and educational attainment. In turn, family roles will influence a woman's employment status and in many cases the nature of her current job (Dex 1984; Brannen *et al.* 1994). These relationships between family roles and structural variables are likely to be substantial for women, but weaker or non-existent for men. The effect of women's family roles on health must be seen within the context of the material resources available to her household and for bringing up children.

As discussed in Chapter 1, there have been profound structural changes in gender roles since the mid-1970s in western societies, leading to the expectation that the pattern of inequalities in health among women and men will also have changed. Women have entered the paid labour force in increasing numbers and many women remain in the role of full-time housewife for only a few years when their children are very young (Brannen *et al.* 1994; Glover and Arber 1995; Hakim 1996). In Britain and many other countries, women have gained greater financial independence, but women and men still occupy different structural locations within society; occupational sex segregation has persisted, and women are more likely to have low incomes (Church 1997).

In the 1990s, a higher proportion of men aged 20–59 are not in paid employment than in the past, because of longer periods of higher education, increased levels of unemployment and earlier age of exit from the labour market (Arber 1997). Fewer people remain in the same occupation for life and an individual's social class may be more likely to change over time. There may be advantages in using socio-economic measures, other than occupational class, which can be applied to all adults and are more stable throughout the lifecourse. These criteria are fulfilled by educational variables, which generally remain fixed after the individual completes full-time education. However, there are cohort differences in the extent and meaning of educational qualifications, with younger age cohorts much more likely to have higher qualifications, such as a degree, than older cohorts (particularly among women). In Britain, educational qualifications have been rarely used in health inequalities research, mainly because of the assumption that a large proportion of the population have no qualifications. However, they have been widely used in other countries, such as the USA (Kitagawa and Hauser 1973) and other parts of Europe, such as Finland (Valkonen 1989; Valkonen *et al.* 1997).

It is timely to reassess the value of educational qualifications in British health inequalities research, especially among women where occupational class may be a less than ideal measure because of occupational downgrading following childbirth (Dex 1984; Brannen *et al.* 1994). Since women and men have a differing relationship to the labour market, it may be that class provides a better measure of inequalities in health for men than for women, whereas educational qualifications provide a better discriminator of health for women.

Within British society, financial and material resources of the household, such as car ownership and housing tenure, are closely tied to success in the labour market. Increasingly for couples, this depends on the labour market position of both partners. In addition, material and financial resources are influenced by state policies, such as eligibility for welfare benefits.

Our attention in this chapter is restricted to examining characteristics of the individual, and not their partner: a fuller discussion of this model is in Arber (1997). The analysis uses logistic regression to examine self-assessed health as 'less than good', based on three years of the GHS (1992–4). We first contrast the association between marital status and self-assessed health for women and men using odds ratios in a model which also controls for five-year age groups (Table 5.2a). Married men and women, the reference category, report better health than any other marital status. Men who are cohabiting report similar health to married men, but cohabiting women report somewhat poorer health than married women. For both sexes, divorced or separated people report the poorest health (odds ratios of 1.59 for men and 1.74 for women). Working age widows and widowers also report poorer health than married people. Since widowed people form a very small proportion of the 20–59 age group, they are combined with divorced and separated people in subsequent analyses. Single men and women have an intermediate level of health, between that of married and previously married people. This contrasts with earlier work which suggested that single women had better health than married women (Verbrugge 1979; Morgan 1980). These analyses by marital status show remarkably similar patterns of

Table 5.2 Odds ratios of 'less than good' health by (a) marital status and (b) family structure, for men and women aged 20–59[1]

	Men Odds ratio	Women Odds ratio	Men		Women	
			%	N	%	N
(a) *Marital status* (Model A)						
Married	1.00	1.00	65.0	10,012	64.9	11,439
Cohabiting	1.07	1.21**	8.3	1,277	7.7	1,357
Single	1.24**	1.37**	20.3	3,128	14.8	2,608
Divorced/separated	1.59**	1.74**	5.7	872	10.3	1,811
Widowed	1.50*	1.48**	0.7	107	2.3	400
N =			100%	15,396	100%	17,615
ΔLLR with marital status	52.2	142.4				
(b) *Family structure* (Model B)						
Married – no children	1.00	1.00	19.3	2,969	20.4	3,588
children in family	1.08	1.03	45.7	7,043	44.6	7,851
Cohabiting – no children	0.96	1.12	5.0	771	4.4	784
children in family	1.41**	1.40**	3.3	506	3.3	573
Single – no children	1.30**	1.16*	20.2	3,113	11.2	1,977
lone parent	1.64	2.32**	0.1	15	3.6	631
Prev. married[2] – no children	1.63**	1.72**	5.0	766	4.7	826
children in family	1.78**	1.73**	1.4	213	7.8	1,385
N =			100%	15,396	100%	17,615
ΔLLR with parental status	63.7	198.4				

Notes: [1] All models include age in five-year age groups
[2] Previously married, includes divorced, separated and widowed people
* Significance of difference from the reference category: * $p < 0.05$; ** $p < 0.01$
Source: General Household Survey 1992/3, 1993/4, 1994/5

health inequalities for women and men of working age. However, it is important to note that women are twice as likely as men to be previously married, 12.6 per cent and 6.4 per cent respectively (final two sets of columns, Table 5.2a), and previous marriage is associated with poor self-assessed health.

To assess the impact of parental roles, we analyse the association between family structure and health for women and men (Table 5.2b) by subdividing each marital status category according to whether children live in their family. Preliminary analyses showed that health patterns were similar for those women with dependent and with grown-up children in the family, so the category 'children in the family' combines these two groups. It is important to note the major gender differences in lone parenthood: 3.6 per cent of women are single mothers and 7.8 per cent are previously married lone mothers. Whereas only 1.4 per cent of men are previously married lone fathers and 0.1 per cent are never married lone fathers.

An interaction between health, marital and parental status is captured by our family structure variable (Table 5.2b). There is no difference in the health of married men and women according to whether or not they have children, and cohabiting men and women with no children report similarly good levels of health; as shown by the odds ratios which are close to 1.00. However, cohabiting men and women with children report significantly poorer health (around odds ratio of 1.40). Single men and women with no children report somewhat poorer health than married people, particularly for men (odds ratios of 1.30). The poorest health is reported by single mothers, who have an odds ratio which is over twice as high (2.32) as married women. Previously married men and women, irrespective of whether they have children, report poorer levels of health than married men and women (odds ratios of 1.72 for women and 1.78 for previously married men with children). Our analyses show that children *per se* have no adverse effect on health, except among single women. The presence of children in the family makes no difference to the health of currently married people, and previously married people report poor health whether or not they have children. However, single women with children are much more likely to report poor health, whereas single women without children show only a small difference from married women. The change in the log likelihood ratio (LLR) shows that family structure explains more of the variance in health for women than for men (a change in LLR of 64 for men and 198 for women for Model B compared to a model which includes only age).

An important issue is to what extent these patterns of health according to family structure can be explained by the varying class or material positions of women and men. Table 5.3 presents nested logistic regression models (in which the small number of never married lone fathers are combined with previously married lone fathers). Model B shows the same odds ratios for family structure as in Table 5.2b. Model C adds educational qualifications and occupational class. Contrasting Model B with Model C shows that part of the poor health reported in some family structures can be explained by education and class, especially for men. For example, the odds ratio of poor health declines from 1.78 to 1.56 for previously married lone fathers once educational qualifications and occupational class are included in Model C. For women the reduction in the effects of family structure are more modest. For never married women, in fact, the odds ratio increases slightly from 1.16 to 1.24 when educational qualifications and occupational class are included in

Table 5.3 Odds ratios of 'less than good' health, men and women aged 20–59[1]

	Men			Women		
	Model B	*Model C*	*Model D*	*Model B*	*Model C*	*Model D*
Family structure	+++	+++	(ns)	+++	+++	++
Married – no children	1.00	1.00	1.00	1.00	1.00	1.00
children in family	1.08	1.03	1.04	1.03	0.96	0.99
Cohabiting – no children	0.96	0.95	0.96	1.12	1.19*	1.23*
children in family	1.41**	1.17	0.99	1.40*	1.27*	1.15
Single – no children	1.30**	1.19**	0.99	1.16*	1.24**	1.10
lone parent	–	–	–	2.32**	1.90**	1.25*
Prev. married – no children	1.63**	1.47**	1.14	1.72**	1.70**	1.27**
children in family	1.78**	1.56**	1.34	1.73**	1.51**	1.16*
Educational qualifications		+++	+++		+++	+++
Degree or professional		1.00	1.00		1.00	1.00
A levels and nursing		1.20**	1.19**		1.19*	1.19*
GCSEs/O levels		1.19**	1.14*		1.35**	1.30**
Commercial/apprentice/CSEs		1.57**	1.47**		1.44**	1.34**
No qualifications		1.79**	1.52**		1.87**	1.54**
Social class		+++	+++		+++	+
High professional/managerial		1.00	1.00		1.00	1.00
Lower professional/managers		1.27**	1.25**		1.22*	1.14
Clerical, routine non-manual		1.29**	1.22*		1.18*	1.09
Skilled manual		1.57**	1.41**		1.23*	1.11
Semi-skilled and unskilled		1.93**	1.54**		1.51**	1.24**
Never worked					2.03**	1.15
Employment status			+++			+++
Full time			1.00			1.00
Part time			1.12			0.96
Unemployed			1.13			1.20*
Keeping house			1.60**			1.33**
Other non-employed			7.70**			5.43**
Car ownership			+++			+++
No car in household			1.00			1.00
One car			0.83**			0.81**
Two or more cars			0.75**			0.71**
Housing tenure			+++			+++
Owner-occupier			1.00			1.00
Private renter			1.15*			1.14*
Local authority/housing assn.			1.35**			1.47**
Model improvement ΔLLR	63.7	426.3	949.5	198.4	316.8	779.4
Change, degrees of freedom	6	8	8	7	9	8
N =	15,396			17,615		

Notes: [1] All models include age in five-year age groups
+ Significance of variable in the model: + p < 0.05; ++ p < 0.01; +++ p < 0.001
* Significance of difference from the reference category: * p < 0.05; ** p < 0.01
Source: General Household Survey 1992/3, 1993/4, 1994/5

Model C, suggesting that single women are on average of a higher class and have more educational qualifications.

Educational qualifications have a strong and linear effect on health for both men and women; those who have no qualifications report the poorest health – odds ratios of 1.79 for men and 1.87 for women in comparison to those with professional qualifications or degrees. Occupational class, measured by the individual's current or last occupation, has a stronger gradient for men than for women, with the odds ratio of poor health increasing by 93 per cent for semi-skilled and unskilled men and 51 per cent for women. Women who have never worked report the poorest health, an odds ratio of 2.03. The change in log likelihood ratio between Model B and Model C (presented at the base of Table 5.3) shows that, unlike family structure, educational qualifications and occupational class explain more of the variance in health for men (change in LLR of 426) than for women (change in LLR of 317).

Model D introduces the structural variables of employment status, housing tenure and car ownership to examine their influence on health inequalities. For men, family structure is no longer statistically significant when these additional structural variables are also included, which suggests that the poorer health of previously married and single men is mainly because of their disadvantaged employment position and material circumstances. For women, family structure remains statistically significant, but most of the odds ratios are now more similar to the reference category of married women. In particular, the odds ratio of poor health for single mothers has fallen dramatically from 2.32 (for Model B), to 1.90 (for Model C) and to 1.25 (for Model D), which suggests that the adverse health of these women is largely because of their lack of paid employment and poor material circumstances (change from Model C to D), as well as their lower level of education and lower occupational class (change from Model B to C). Similarly for previously married women it has fallen sharply, for example from 1.51 (Model C) to 1.16 (Model D) for those with children.

Occupational class for women becomes a less important predictor of poor health, once employment status and the two indicators of material circumstances are included in the model, but educational qualifications remain highly statistically significant. For men, both educational qualifications and occupational class remain highly significant predictors of self-assessed health. Women who care for the home full time have a third higher odds of poor health than women working full time, and women who are unemployed have a significantly increased odds ratio of poor health. The small number of men who say they care for the home full time have an odds ratio of 1.60. There is surprisingly little evidence of poorer health among unemployed men. However, both men and women who are non-employed for other reasons (e.g. early retired and disabled people) report particularly poor health. It is likely that unemployed people with poor health in the 1990s leave the labour market and define themselves as non-employed for other reasons, such as disability (Bartley and Owen 1996).

The two measures of material circumstances, housing tenure and car ownership, are associated with health in similar ways for women and men. Those in households with cars report better health, and those living in local authority (or housing association) properties report poorer health than owner-occupiers, after class, education and employment status have been controlled for in the models.

In sum, our analysis has shown that both educational qualifications and social class, based on the individual's own occupation, are closely associated with self-assessed health. Men and women whose current or last job is in a lower class occupation and who have less educational qualifications are most likely to report poor health. These patterns are broadly similar for men and women, although there is a weaker class gradient for women, whereas the gradient with educational qualifications is comparable for women and men.

Our analyses suggest that changes in family structure since the 1970s, particularly the growth in lone parenthood and cohabitation, need to be taken into account when analysing gender differences in health inequalities. The previous orthodoxy that married women have poorer health than single women no longer holds, possibly reflecting changes in the meaning of marriage in the late twentieth century and career opportunities for married women which in the late 1960s were viable only for single women. Parenthood in disadvantaged material circumstances is a determinant of poor health, especially for single mothers. We have shown that single mothers and divorced and separated people in the 1990s report particularly poor self-assessed health, which can be explained largely by their disadvantaged structural circumstances.

The growth of unemployment and increases in income inequality since the late 1970s, plus increases in divorce and lone parenthood, suggest that more direct measures of structural position in addition to occupational social class are needed. Including educational attainment, employment status and family structure provides a more adequate framework for understanding inequalities in health.

Later life

Many studies of class inequalities in health omit the population above working age. Two factors highlight the need to consider this group in studies of health inequalities: first, the growth in the proportion of the population above state pension age; and second, the earlier age at which both men and women leave paid employment in western societies (Kohli *et al.* 1991). The expectation of life for women in Britain is 79 and for men is 74 (ONS 1998). The time between labour market exit and death is increasing, averaging 17 years for men and 22 years for women in Britain. It is ironic that so little research attention has been paid to inequalities in health among men and women in later life, despite the increasing proportion of adult life spent after leaving paid work.

The current generation of older British women have had a very different lifecourse from that of older men. Many of these older women left the labour market when they got married or had children, and either did not return to paid employment or returned to part-time rather than full-time work once their children were older (Dex 1984). Thus marital and parental status will have had a profound effect on the lifecourse of the current cohort of older women, especially regarding participation in paid employment. As well as serving in the Second World War, this generation of older men have experienced full employment for most of their lives, apart from some of the oldest old who were of working age during the Depression of the late 1920s and early 1930s.

A major gender difference in later life relates to marital status. In Britain, half of women over the age of 65 are widowed, whereas this is the case for only 17 per cent of men, while 71 per cent of older men are married, compared to 39 per cent of older women (ONS 1998). Only 4 per cent of the current cohort of older women and men are divorced. The latter proportion will increase for future generations of older people, as a consequence of the high divorce rates of the 1980s and 1990s. We expect from previous research that married older people in the 1990s will report better self-assessed health than previously married people (Morgan 1980; Anson 1989). However, when using surveys of people living in private households, it is relevant to bear in mind that marital status influences the likelihood of entry into residential or institutional care among older people (Arber and Cooper 1999). Those who have never married are most likely to live in a residential setting followed by widowed and divorced people, with much lower proportions among married people. Glaser and Grundy (1997) analysed limiting longstanding illness using data from the 1991 Population Census in Britain and found that the health of never married older people in community samples is better than married people, but this is *not* the case if older people resident in institutions are included in the analysis.

A key concern is to what extent occupational class continues to structure the health inequalities of men and women in later life. As we noted earlier, the class of married women has often been measured by their husband's occupation (Goldthorpe 1983), but among older women only a minority are married. Therefore for most older women, the only option is to measure class based on their last occupation, which for the current generation of older women may have been before marriage, many years earlier. Earlier work in Britain (Arber and Ginn 1991, 1993) and comparable research in Finland (Rahkonen and Takala 1998) and in Norway (Dahl and Birkelund 1997) shows strong class inequalities in health among older men and women. Here we examine inequalities in older women's and men's health in the 1990s according to class, income and housing tenure. We expect that the continuing influence of class based on older people's position in the labour market during their working life will be less for older women than for older men.

The concentration of poverty among women is particularly marked in later life (Arber and Ginn 1991; Ginn and Arber 1996). Income inequalities among the older population have increased since the late 1970s, leading to income polarization between those with a good occupational pension and those reliant only on a state pension (Evandrou 1997). Two-thirds of British women aged over 65 have to rely solely on state pensions, and are therefore in poverty, whereas this is the case for one-third of older men (Ginn and Arber 1999b). Since occupational pension income in later life is to a considerable extent related to position in the labour market during working life, especially for men, it is important to analyse the effects of income on health after controlling for occupational class within the same model.

We use the General Household Survey for three years (1992–4) to consider briefly gender differences in health in later life before examining structural inequalities in health among older men and women. There is little gender difference in the proportion of older men and women who assess their health as 'less than good' under age 80. Above age 80, 70 per cent of women and 64 per cent of men report 'less than good' health, compared to 54 per cent of both men and women aged 65–9. The small gender difference in self-assessed health contrasts markedly with the substantial gender difference in functional impairment in later life (Arber and Cooper 1999).

Despite the modest gender differences in self-assessed health in later life, health inequalities according to class are very striking at all ages among older men and women, see Figure 5.3. In each five-year age group under 80, about 30 per cent *more* men previously in a professional occupation rate their health as 'good' than men previously in a semi- or unskilled occupation, while 20 per cent *more* professional men than semi- and unskilled men report their health as 'good' even in their 80s. Social class differences are so strong and consistent that differences in self-reported health by age are much less important than differences by class; for example, fewer men in their late 60s who previously worked in manual

Figure 5.3 Percentage reporting good health by socio-economic group, men and women aged 65+

Men

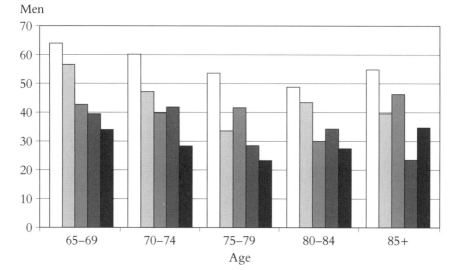

Women

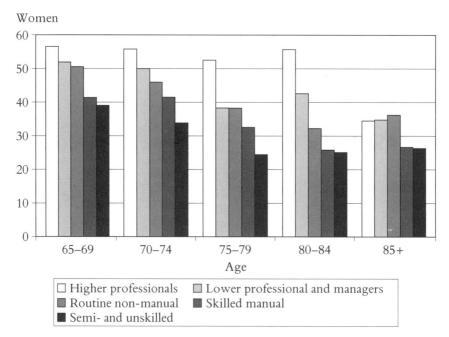

☐ Higher professionals   ▨ Lower professional and managers
▨ Routine non-manual   ▨ Skilled manual
■ Semi- and unskilled

Source: General Household Survey 1992/3, 1993/4, 1994/5

occupations rate their health as 'good' than professional men twenty years their senior. For older women, class gradients in self-assessed health are also linear and consistent across the age range. However, they are somewhat weaker among women than men in some age groups.

These very strong and consistent class differences in self-assessed health indicate the resilience of social class during working life in influencing health into very old age. Although class differences in survival mean one would expect a reduction in class inequalities in health with advancing age, this does not occur, except for women in their late 80s.

Class inequalities in self-assessed health are further examined using logistic regression (see Table 5.4). Model A shows that occupational class has a statistically significant effect on self-assessed health in later life when marital status and age are included in the model. The gradients are strong, with men previously in semi-skilled and unskilled occupations having nearly three times higher odds of poor health compared with professional/managerial men, while for women the odds ratios are over twice as high for women who previously worked in semi-skilled and unskilled occupations. It is remarkable that older women's own occupational class has such a significant effect on their health, as a weaker gradient between class and health was expected. Older women who have never worked (about 6 per cent of women aged 65 and over) also report poorer health than those previously in professional or managerial occupations.

Despite the variation in marital status between older women and men, and the differences in health by marital status reported earlier for working age adults, marital status does not have a statistically significant effect on self-assessed health for either older women or men. The odds ratios of poor health for the married and widowed are similar, but are somewhat higher for older divorced/separated women. The general lack of a marital status effect may be partly due to the selective effect of marital status on entry into residential care, as discussed earlier.

Our analysis includes household income, measured in quintiles after equivalizing for the number of adults in the household, and this is strongly associated with self-reported health (Table 5.4, Model B). Older women and men with the highest 20 per cent of income report the best health (the reference category), with little difference between the self-assessed health of other income groups. A similar pattern is seen for older women and men; those in the lower 60 per cent of the income distribution have their odds ratios of poor health increased by approximately 60 per cent.

Housing tenure is also significantly associated with self-reported health for both sexes. Older people living in local authority housing have higher odds of reporting poor health than owner-occupiers. It is possible that the housing tenure difference partly reflects reverse causation.

Table 5.4   Odds ratios of 'less than good' health, men and women aged 65+[1]

	Men		Women	
	Model A	*Model B*	*Model A*	*Model B*
Marital status	ns	ns	ns	ns
Married	1.00	1.00	1.00	1.00
Single	1.22	1.17	0.94	0.90
Widowed	1.13	1.10	1.00	0.94
Divorced/separated	1.25	1.10	1.37★	1.17
Social class	+++	+++	+++	+++
Professional/managerial	1.00	1.00	1.00	1.00
Routine non-manual	1.59★★★	1.42★★	1.26★★	1.17
Skilled manual	1.97★★★	1.51★★★	1.69★★★	1.39★★
Semi-/unskilled	2.75★★★	1.99★★★	2.06★★★	1.58★★★
Never worked			1.91★★★	1.82★★★
Household income		+++		+++
Highest 20%		1.00		1.00
60 < 80%		1.42★★★		1.49★★★
40 < 60%		1.57★★★		1.66★★★
20 < 40%		1.58★★★		1.66★★★
Lowest 20%		1.60★★★		1.54★★★
Length of current housing tenure		+++		+++
Owner-occupier 5+ years		1.00		1.00
Owner-occupier <5 years		1.02		1.02
Private renter		0.95		0.91
Local authority 5+ years		1.48★★★		1.65★★★
Local authority <5 years		1.62★★★		1.85★★★
N =	3,985		5,624	
Δ LLR (Δ df)	130.9 (6)	64.4 (8)	101.1 (7)	132.2 (8)

Notes: [1] Model also includes age in five-year age groups
   ★ Significance of difference from the reference category: ★ $p < 0.05$; ★★ $p < 0.01$;
   ★★★ $p < 0.001$
   + Significance of variable in the model: + $p < 0.05$; ++ $p < 0.01$; +++ $p < 0.001$
Source: General Household Survey 1992/3, 1993/4, 1994/5

For example, an older person might have moved to local authority sheltered housing because of increased disability. However, Table 5.4 subdivides the two main housing tenures according to whether the older person had moved in the previous five years, and found little evidence that those who had recently moved reported poorer health.

Our analyses show that income has a similar effect on self-assessed health for both sexes, but previous occupational class has a stronger effect on health for older men than for older women, which can be seen from the greater change in log likelihood ratios (LLR) for men than for women for Model A. Whereas the change in LLR is greater for women than men in Model B, when income and housing tenure are included. The poorer health of divorced/separated older women is no longer evident when income and housing tenure are included in Model B, which suggests that the disadvantaged health of these older women relates to their poor material circumstances.

The similarity of the pattern of inequalities in health for older women and men is surprising given the very marked differences in the lifecourse of older women and men, the majority of these women having spent less than half of their adult life in paid employment. It is likely that the next generation of older men and women will show even greater similarity in the pattern of health disadvantage according to class and other structural variables. Our findings demonstrate that similar structural factors are associated with poor health in later life as during working life and that earlier lifecourse, particularly position in the occupational structure, has a major continuing influence on health even among the oldest old. A person's last main occupation during working life provides a good measure of class position in later life. However, the current high divorce rate may have implications for the next generation of older people, resulting in poorer health for older divorced women who have lived much of their life in disadvantaged material circumstances.

Conclusion

This chapter has examined the extent to which there are similarities and differences between men and women in the pattern of health inequalities during childhood, the working ages and later life. We have shown comparable patterns of health inequalities for boys and girls in childhood. In this period of the lifecourse, employment status of the parents is a more important factor influencing levels of chronic illness than social class of their family head.

During the working ages, there are gender differences in the pattern of health inequalities with family structure having a greater effect on women's than on men's health. Married men and women report the best health, irrespective of whether they have children. Single mothers report much poorer health than married women and men. Social class continues to be a major factor determining the health of working age men and women. However, it is important to take into account other structural variables, which have been of increasing salience since the late 1990s. Whether or not a person is in paid employment is now a key marker of health status, and educational qualifications increasingly differentiate health in the working age group, especially among women. A multivariate approach to understanding inequalities in health is advocated, which simultaneously examines a number of variables relating to family structure (marital and parental status), structural position (such as class, educational qualifications and employment status) and material resources (such as housing tenure and car ownership).

Among the current generation of older British men and women there are strong class differences in health, and remarkable similarities in the pattern of health inequalities for older men and women. As stated earlier, major historical social changes experienced by the current cohort of older people mean that these gender differences in the pattern of health inequalities may differ for later cohorts who enter retirement in the twenty-first century.

This chapter has used research data from the 1990s drawn from large British surveys. It must be borne in mind that a different picture would emerge if data were analysed for earlier or later historical time periods. The nature of inequalities in women's and men's health is likely to differ over time and between societies in concert with the way in which gender roles and relationships vary historically and cross-nationally. In taking a lifecourse approach, we have provided added insights into the mechanisms underlying the creation and perpetuation of health inequalities in 1990s Britain. We have argued that although class remains an important indicator of inequalities in health, the current emphasis on social class may be masking other important dimensions of inequality relating to an individual's structural position and family circumstances. Continued reliance on social class measures may also underestimate the extent of inequalities in women's health, which may be more saliently captured using measures of educational level and family structure.

Acknowledgements

We are grateful to the Office for National Statistics for permission to use data from the General Household Survey, and to the Data Archive and Manchester Computing Centre for access to the data. We particularly appreciate the helpful comments of Jay Ginn on an earlier draft of this chapter and those of the editors.

References

Acheson Report (1998) *Independent Inquiry into Inequalities in Health Report.* Chairman: Sir Donald Acheson. London: Stationery Office.

Anson, O. (1989) Marital status and women's health revisited: the importance of a proximate adult, *Journal of Marriage and the Family*, 51: 185–94.

Arber, S. (1989) Gender and class inequalities in health: understanding the differentials, in A. J. Fox (ed.) *Inequalities in Health in European Countries*. Aldershot: Gower.

Arber, S. (1991) Class, paid employment and family roles: making sense of structural disadvantage, gender and health status, *Social Science and Medicine*, 32(4): 425–36.

Arber, S. (1997) Comparing inequalities in women's and men's health: Britain in the 1990s, *Social Science and Medicine*, 44(6): 773–87.

Arber, S. and Cooper, H. (1999) Gender differences in health in later life: the new paradox?, *Social Science and Medicine*, 48(1): 61–76.

Arber, S. and Evandrou, M. (eds) (1993) *Ageing, Independence and the Life Course*. London: Jessica Kingsley.

Arber, S. and Ginn, J. (1991) *Gender and Later Life: A Sociological Analysis of Resources and Constraints*. London: Sage.

Arber, S. and Ginn, J. (1993) Gender and inequalities in health in later life, *Social Science and Medicine*, 34(1): 33–44.

Arber, S. and Ginn, J. (1995) *Connecting Gender and Ageing: A Sociological Approach*. Buckingham: Open University Press.

Arber, S., Gilbert, G. N. and Dale, A. (1985) Paid employment and women's health: a benefit or a source of role strain?, *Sociology of Health and Illness*, 7(3): 377–400.

Bartley, M. and Owen, C. (1996) Relation between socioeconomic status, employment and health during economic change, 1973–93, *British Medical Journal*, 313: 445–9.

Bartley, M., Popay, J. and Plewis, I. (1992) Domestic conditions, paid employment and women's experience of ill health, *Sociology of Health and Illness*, 14(3): 313–43.

Bennett, N., Jarvis, L., Rowlands, O., Singleton, N. and Haselden, L. (1996) *Living in Britain: Results of the 1994 General Household Survey*. London: HMSO.

Brannen, J., Meszaros, G., Moss, P. and Poland, G. (1994) *Employment and Family Life: A Review of Research in the UK*. London: Department of Employment.

Buck, N., Gershuny, J., Rose, D. and Scott, J. (1994) *Changing Households: The British Household Panel Survey 1990–92*. Colchester: ESRC Research Centre on Micro-social Change.

Church, J. (ed.) (1997) *Social Trends 27*. Office for National Statistics. London: HMSO.

Cooper, H., Arber, S. and Smaje, C. (1998) Social class or deprivation? Structural factors and children's limiting longstanding illness in the 1990s, *Sociology of Health and Illness*, 20(3): 289–311.

Dahl, E. and Birkelund, G. E. (1997) Health inequalities in later life in a social democratic welfare state, *Social Science and Medicine*, 44(6): 859–970.

Dale, A. (1995) The changing context of childhood: demographic and economic changes, in B. Botting (ed.) *The Health of Our Children: Decennial Supplement*, OPCS, DS no. 11. London: HMSO.

Dex, S. (1984) *Women's Work Histories: An Analysis of the Women and Employment Survey*, Department of Employment research paper no. 46. London: DoE.

Drever, F. and Whitehead, M. (eds) (1997) *Health Inequalities, Decennial Supplement*. Office for National Statistics, DS no. 15. London: Stationery Office.

Evandrou, M. (ed.) (1997) *Baby Boomers: Ageing in the 21st Century*. London: Age Concern.

Fogelman, K. (ed.) (1983) *Growing Up in Great Britain: Papers from the National Child Development Study*. London: Macmillan.

Ginn, J. and Arber, S. (1996) Patterns of employment, pensions and gender: the effect of work history on older women's non-state pensions, *Work, Employment and Society*, 10(3): 469–90.

Ginn, J. and Arber, S. (1998) How does part-time work lead to low pension income?, in J. O'Reilly and C. Fagan (eds) *Part-time Prospects: An International Comparison of Part-time Work in Europe, North America and the Pacific Rim*. London: Routledge.

Ginn, J. and Arber, S. (1999a) Gender, the generational contract and pension privatisation, in S. Arber and C. Attias-Donfut (eds) *The Myth of Generational Conflict: The Family and State in Ageing Societies*. European Sociological Association series. London: Routledge.

Ginn, J. and Arber, S. (1999b) Women's pension poverty: prospects and options for change, in S. Walby (ed.) *New Agendas for Women*. London: Macmillan.

Glaser, K. and Grundy, E. (1997) Marital status and long-term illness in Great Britain, *Journal of Marriage and the Family*, 59: 156–64.

Glover, J. and Arber, S. (1995) Polarisation in mother's employment: Occupational class, age of youngest child, employment rights and work hours, *Gender, Work and Organisation*, 2(4): 165–79.

Goldthorpe, J. (1983) Women and class analysis: in defence of the conventional view, *Sociology*, 17(4): 465–87.

Hakim, C. (1996) *Key Issues in Women's Work: Female Heterogeneity and Polarisaton of Women's Employment*. London: Athlone.

Idler, E. L. and Benyamini, Y. (1997) Self-rated health and mortality: a review of twenty-seven community studies, *Journal of Health and Social Behaviour*, 38: 21–37.

Kiernan, K. and Estaugh, E. (1993) *Cohabitation*. London: Family Policy Studies Centre.

Kitagawa, E. M. and Hauser, P. M. (1973) *Differential Mortality in the United States: A Study of Socioeconomic Epidemiology*. Cambridge, MA: Harvard University Press.

Kohli, M., Rein, M., Guillemard, A-M. and van Gunsteren, H. (eds) (1991) *Time for Retirement: Comparative Studies of Early Exit from the Labour Force*. Cambridge: Cambridge University Press.

Lahelma, E. and Rahkonen, O. (1997) Health inequalities in modern societies and beyond, special issue of *Social Science and Medicine*, 44(6): 721–910.

Laslett, P. (1989) *A Fresh Map of Life*. London: Weidenfeld and Nicolson.

Macran, S., Clarke, L., Sloggett, A. and Bethune, A. (1994) Women's socio-economic status and self-assessed health: identifying some disadvantaged groups, *Sociology of Health and Illness*, 16(2): 182–208.

Macran, S., Clarke, L. and Joshi, H. (1996) Women's health: dimensions and differentials, *Social Science and Medicine*, 42(9): 1203–16.

Mannheim, K. (1952) The problem of generations, in K. Mannheim, *Essays on the Sociology of Knowledge*. London: Routledge and Kegan Paul.

Morgan, M. (1980) Marital status, health, illness and service use, *Social Science and Medicine*, 14A(6): 633–43.

Mossey, J. M. and Shapiro, E. (1982) Self-rated health: a predictor of mortality among the elderly, *American Journal of Public Health*, 72: 800–8.

Nathanson, C. (1980) Social roles and health status among women: the significance of employment, *Social Science and Medicine*, 14A(6): 463–71.

Office for National Statistics (ONS) (1998) *Population Trends 94*. London: Stationery Office.

Popay, J. and Jones, G. (1990) Patterns of health and illness amongst lone parents, *Journal of Social Policy*, 19(4): 499–534.

Power, C., Manor, O. and Fox, J. (1993) *Health and Class: The Early Years*. London: Chapman Hall.

Rahkonen, O. and Takala, P. (1998) Social class differences in health and functional disability among older men and women, *International Journal of Health Services*, 28(3): 511–24.

Sweeting, H. and West, P. (1995) Family life and health in adolescence: a role for culture in the health inequalities debate?, *Social Science and Medicine*, 40(2): 163–75.

Townsend, P. and Davidson, N. (1982) *Inequalities in Health: The Black Report*. Harmondsworth: Penguin.

Valkonen, T. (1989) Adult mortality and level of education: a comparison of six countries, in A. J. Fox (ed.) *Health Inequalities in European Countries*. Aldershot: Gower.

Valkonen, T., Sihvonen, A. and Lahelma, E. (1997) Health expectancy by level of education in Finland, *Social Science and Medicine*, 44(6): 801–8.

Verbrugge, L. (1979) Marital status and health, *Journal of Marriage and the Family*, 41: 267–85.

Verbrugge, L. (1983) Multiple roles and physical health of women and men, *Journal of Health and Social Behavior*, 24: 16–30.

Wadsworth, M. (1997) Health inequalities in the life course perspective, *Social Science and Medicine*, 44(6): 859–70.

West, P. (1988) Inequalities? Social class differentials in health in British youth, *Social Science and Medicine*, 27(4): 291–6.

West, P. (1997) Health inequalities in the early years: is there equalisation in youth?, *Social Science and Medicine*, 44(6): 833–58.

West, P., Macintyre, S., Annandale, E. and Hunt, K. (1990) Social class and health in youth: findings from the West of Scotland Twenty-07 Study, *Social Science and Medicine*, 30(6): 665–73.

Wilkinson, R. (1996) *Unhealthy Societies: The Afflictions of Inequality*. London: Routledge.

Wyke, S. and Ford, G. (1992) Competing explanations for associations between marital status and health, *Social Science and Medicine*, 34(5): 525–32.

six

Trends in gender differences in mortality: relationships to changing gender differences in behaviour and other causal factors

Ingrid Waldron

Introduction

It is well known that males have higher mortality than females for total mortality and for most causes of death in contemporary developed countries. Males' higher mortality is due in large part to gender differences in health related behaviour (for example, males' higher rates of cigarette smoking and heavy drinking) and biological factors (for example, effects of sex hormones on ischaemic heart disease risk) (Gee and Veevers 1983; Lopez 1983; United Nations 1988; Waldron 1995a, 1995b).

Gender differences in mortality have varied historically. In developed countries, gender differences in mortality generally increased during the mid-twentieth century, because females had more favourable mortality trends than males (Enterline 1961; Preston 1976; United Nations 1982; Gee and Veevers 1983; Lopez 1983; United Nations 1988; Waldron 1993). For example, sex mortality ratios (the male death rate divided by the female death rate) generally increased during the mid-twentieth century; sex mortality ratios increased because female mortality decreased proportionately more than male mortality. The trend to increasing gender differences ended around 1980 in the USA and some other developed countries (United Nations 1988; Waldron 1993, 1995a; Trovato and Lalu 1998). For example, during the 1980s in the USA, sex mortality ratios decreased somewhat, as males experienced proportionately greater decreases in mortality than females.

This chapter analyses US data for 1950–90 to describe trends in male and female mortality and the resulting trends in sex mortality ratios. Trends are described for total mortality and for several major causes of death which have large gender differences, specifically, lung cancer, ischaemic heart disease, motor vehicle accidents, other accidents, suicide and homicide. This chapter also investigates the causes of these trends in death rates and sex mortality ratios. Previous research has shown that gender differences in health related behaviour are a major cause of gender differences in mortality, so trends in male and female health related behaviour are investigated in this chapter (Gee and Veevers 1983; Lopez 1983; Waldron 1995a). Investigators of socio-economic differentials in health and mortality have emphasized the importance of structural/ materialist factors such as housing conditions; however, structural/ materialist factors appear to make a much smaller contribution to gender differences in mortality, and therefore will receive relatively little atten- tion (Waldron 1991a, 1995a; Stronks *et al.* 1996). For convenience, the term 'behaviour' is used inclusively to refer to a broad range of be- haviours, including typical health related behaviours such as smoking and behaviours which influence structural/materialist factors, such as working in a particular occupation. In order to investigate whether the trends observed in the USA may generalize to other developed countries, US mortality trends are briefly compared to trends in other Anglophone countries and western European countries.

At a descriptive level, this chapter addresses several questions. For each cause of death, have death rates decreased or increased? Have males and females experienced similar proportionate changes in mortality, resulting in stable sex mortality ratios? For which causes of death and which time periods have males experienced more favourable mortality trends than females, resulting in decreasing sex mortality ratios? Con- versely, in which cases have females experienced more favourable mort- ality trends, resulting in increasing sex mortality ratios? Each type of trend would be predicted on the basis of one or more of the causal hypotheses presented in the next section.

Hypotheses

The first hypothesis proposes that many of the factors which influence mortality have similar effects on males and females, so males and females tend to have similar mortality trends, and consequently sex mortality ratios tend to be stable. Previous analyses of international and historical data provide mixed support for this hypothesis, with highly correlated variation in male and female death rates for some causes of death in some time periods, but not in other cases (Preston 1976; Waldron 1993, 1995b).

The remaining hypotheses propose several interrelated causes of changes in gender differences in mortality. One hypothesis proposes that trends in gender differences in cigarette smoking have been a major cause of trends in gender differences in mortality. Considerable evidence supports this hypothesis. Men's earlier and more widespread adoption of cigarette smoking was a major contributor to increasing male lung cancer and ischaemic heart disease mortality, which in turn were major contributors to increasing gender differences in total mortality during the mid-twentieth century (Lopez 1983; United Nations 1988). More recently, gender differences in smoking have decreased, and this has contributed to decreasing gender differences in lung cancer, chronic obstructive pulmonary disease, and total mortality during the 1980s in the USA and some other countries (Waldron 1993; Koskinen *et al.* 1994–5; Waldron 1995a). Thus, trends in gender differences in cigarette smoking have had multiple important effects on trends in gender differences in mortality. However, as discussed below, other factors have also had an important influence on trends in gender differences in mortality during the 1950–90 study period.

Another hypothesis proposes that decreasing gender differences in labour force participation rates have resulted in decreasing gender differences in health related behaviour and mortality. This hypothesis proposes that women who are employed experience increased mortality risk because they are exposed to occupational hazards and job stresses. In addition, this hypothesis proposes that employed women are more prone to adopt risky behaviours, such as heavy drinking or smoking, due to increased independence and personal income and the influence of co-workers. Current evidence provides little support for this hypothesis. In contemporary developed countries, labour force participation appears to have only weak and mixed effects on women's health related behaviour and mortality (Waldron 1991a, 1991b, 1997). Also, analyses of trends in gender differences indicate that recent trends in gender differences in labour force participation have had little effect on trends in gender differences in health related behaviour or mortality (Waldron 1991b, 1993, 1995a, 1997).

A related hypothesis, the Women's Emancipation Hypothesis, proposes that the changing roles of women and a general liberalization of norms concerning women's behaviour have resulted in decreasing gender differences in health related behaviour and, consequently, decreasing gender differences in mortality (Waldron 1997; Trovato and Lalu 1998). As discussed in the previous paragraph, women's labour force participation appears to have little direct effect on their health related behaviour and mortality. However, the Women's Emancipation Hypothesis suggests that increases in women's labour force participation may have had indirect effects on trends in women's health related behaviour; specifically, increased employment of women appears to have contributed to a general shift in cultural norms, with a general relaxation of restrictions on women's behaviour. In accord with this hypothesis, during the mid-twentieth century in the USA, decreases in social disapproval of women's smoking contributed to increases in women's smoking and decreases in gender differences in smoking, and these trends contributed to subsequent decreases in gender differences in mortality for lung cancer and chronic obstructive pulmonary disease (Burbank 1972; Waldron 1991b, 1995a). However, contrary to the predictions of the Women's Emancipation Hypothesis, gender differences for many other types of health related behaviour have not decreased in recent decades (based on US data from the 1960s through to the early 1970s; Waldron 1997).

I have proposed a new hypothesis which attempts to account for the varied trends in gender differences for different types of health related behaviour (Waldron 1997). The Gender Roles Modernization Hypothesis proposes that fundamental aspects of traditional gender roles have interacted with recent changes in socio-economic, cultural and material conditions to influence behavioural trends during the 1950–90 study period. Women's traditional focus on care of the family continues to be important in the contemporary USA, but, from the 1950s through to the 1990s, there has been a trend for women's family care to involve less direct childcare and housework and more employment in order to provide financial resources (Bianchi 1995; Robinson and Godbey 1997). Similarly, men's traditional focus on earning an income continues to be important, but 1965–85 data indicate a trend for men to spend less time in employment and more time in housework. These data also indicate that time devoted to childcare showed similar proportionate decreases for both men and women (Robinson and Godbey 1997). This trend reflects the combined effects of decreased childbearing, increased proportions of children who live with their mothers only, and changes in time allocation by parents who live with children. In summary, gender differences in time devoted to employment and housework have decreased, but there appears to have been little change in gender differences in time devoted to childcare, which continues to be primarily the responsibility of women. Thus, fundamental aspects of traditional gender roles continue to influence men's and women's activities, but changes in economic context and attitudes have resulted in substantial reductions in gender differences in some activities.

The Gender Roles Modernization Hypothesis postulates that, similarly, trends in gender differences in health related behaviour have been influenced by the interacting effects of fundamental aspects of traditional gender roles and contemporary conditions. One specific prediction is that women are more likely to adopt health related behaviours which are seen as compatible with fundamental aspects of traditional female roles. For example, in the contemporary USA women's driving serves many functions for the family, so this hypothesis predicts increases in women's driving and decreases in gender differences in driving. In contrast, heavy drinking may interfere with a woman's ability to meet traditional female responsibilities for childcare and sexual restraint, and thus women are not expected to adopt heavy drinking and gender differences in heavy drinking are not expected to decrease.

Other interactions between traditional gender roles and contemporary circumstances may also have influenced recent trends in gender differences in health related behaviour. For example, traditional gender roles encourage women to be more concerned than men with preserving health, so women are predicted to respond more to public health campaigns, such as recent campaigns in the USA to improve diet, to increase exercise and seatbelt use, and to decrease smoking or drinking and driving. This argument leads to the prediction that gender differences in health related behaviour may increase in response to public health campaigns. In addition, contemporary changes in male and female family roles may affect trends in gender differences in health related behaviour. For example, parents who live with children may avoid risky behaviours, so increases in the proportion of men who do not live with their children may tend to increase men's risky behaviour, resulting in increased gender differences in risky behaviour (Umberson 1987; Waldron and Lye 1989; Robinson and Godbey 1997).

In summary, the Gender Roles Modernization Hypothesis proposes that recent trends in gender differences in behaviour have been influenced by the interacting effects of fundamental aspects of traditional gender roles and the contemporary context. These causal factors are predicted to result in varied trends in gender differences for different types of health related behaviour; these behavioural trends in turn are predicted to contribute to varied trends in gender differences for different causes of death. Preliminary investigations have provided some support for the predictions of this hypothesis (Waldron 1995a, 1997).

The final hypothesis proposes that trends in gender differences in mortality have been influenced by multiple diverse factors, in addition to trends in health related behaviour. Evidence related to this and the previous hypotheses is presented in subsequent sections on mortality trends for specific causes of death in the USA. It will be seen that mortality trends have been very different for different causes of death and different time periods, reflecting the wide variety of causal factors which have influenced these mortality trends. In the conclusion to this chapter, the evidence concerning the diverse patterns observed for the specific causes of death is synthesized in discussions of each of the causal hypotheses presented above.

Analysis of mortality trends

Data and methods

Age-adjusted death rates for the USA for 1950–92 were obtained from published sources or calculated from published data (National Center for Health Statistics 1953–94, 1973, 1974, 1978, 1978–95; Grove and Hetzel 1968). To avoid excessive complexity, age and ethnic differences in trends are not discussed in this chapter; these differences have been discussed in previous analyses (e.g. Enterline 1961; Gee and Veevers 1983; Trovato and Lalu 1998; Waldron 1998a, 1998b).

Each cause of death analysed in this study had a sex mortality ratio of 2.0 or more and accounted for at least 1 per cent of deaths in the USA. Among the nine specific causes of death which met these criteria in 1989, the six included in this study were chosen because they had particularly high death rates and/or behavioural interest and reasonably comparable death rate data over the whole study period (Waldron 1995a). Chronic obstructive pulmonary disease was excluded due to lack of comparable data over the study period, and HIV/AIDS, chronic liver disease and cirrhosis were excluded due to relatively low death rates.

During the time period covered, death rates have been coded according to four different International Classifications of Diseases (ICD 6 for 1950–7; ICD 7 for 1958–67; ICD 8 for 1968–78; ICD 9 for 1979–92). Changes in the coding of causes of death had relatively minor effects on the trends described in this chapter, except for ischaemic heart disease (National Center for Health Statistics 1953–94, 1978, 1980). In 1968, the change in ICD coding resulted in the inclusion of more deaths in the ischaemic heart disease category, and these deaths tended to be disproportionately female. The change in ICD coding in 1979 had approximately the reverse effect. To reduce the effects of these changes, ischaemic heart disease death rates for 1968–78 have been multiplied by the appropriate comparability ratio in order to make the 1970s death rates more comparable to the 1980s death rates. For each cause of death, the data presented in the figures represent average death rates over successive intervals, approximately five years each, but restricted to time periods within a single ICD coding; these intervals, together with the designations used in the figures, are 1950–3 = 1951, 1954–7 = 1955, 1958–62 = 1960, 1963–7 = 1965, 1968–72 = 1970, 1973–8 = 1975, 1979–82 = 1980, 1983–7 = 1985 and 1988–92 = 1990.

In order to show how trends have varied during different parts of the 40-year study interval, the mortality data are presented in graphs. Female death rates are plotted on the X axis and male death rates on the Y axis. In these graphs, points with the same sex mortality ratio fall on a straight line, since male death rate = sex mortality ratio × female death rate. Relevant sex mortality ratio lines are shown on the graphs, so trends in sex mortality ratios can be estimated from the figures. The text provides exact sex mortality ratios for individual years of interest.

Data concerning trends in health related behaviour were derived from national surveys of adults and older teenagers. The smoking prevalence data for 1965 and later are age adjusted, but other behavioural data presented are not age adjusted. The sources of the behavioural data presented in the figure are as follows: prevalence of smoking and heavy drinking (US Department of Health and Human Services 1980; Schoenborn 1988; National Center for Health Statistics 1992, 1995; Piani and Schoenborn 1993) and proportion with a driving licence (Veevers 1982; US Department of Transportation 1993). Beginning in the 1980s for smoking and the mid-1970s for heavy drinking, estimates of prevalence have been averaged over five-year intervals to provide greater stability and clarity of the data in the figure. Gender differences in health related behaviours have been assessed with sex ratios, corresponding to the sex mortality ratios used to assess gender differences in mortality.

Lung cancer

In the USA, lung cancer mortality increased for both males and females during the study period, 1950–90. During the early part of this period, lung cancer mortality increased more rapidly for males, so sex mortality ratios increased (Figure 6.1; Burbank 1972; Lopez 1983). Conversely, during the later part of the period, lung cancer mortality increased more rapidly for females, so sex mortality ratios decreased (Figure 6.1; Waldron 1995a). Thus, sex mortality ratios for lung cancer increased from 4.6 in 1950 to a maximum of 6.7 in 1960, and then decreased to 2.3 in 1990.

Previous analyses indicate that these trends in lung cancer mortality have been largely due to trends in cigarette smoking, with a lag of approximately two to three decades between cigarette smoke exposure

Figure 6.1 Trends in male and female mortality for lung cancer, ischaemic heart disease and total mortality, USA, 1950–90

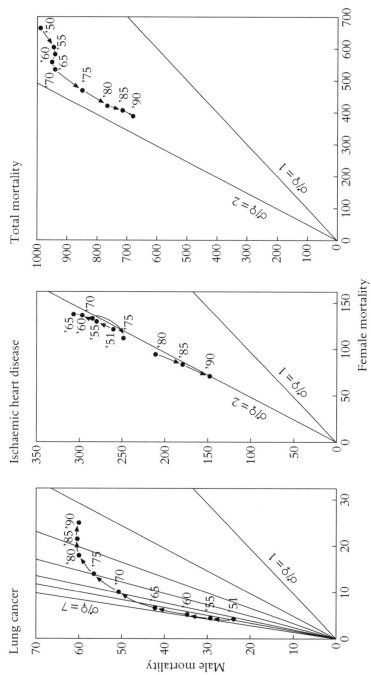

Note: Male and female mortality are shown as age-adjusted death rates per hundred thousand population. Note that scales differ for the different component graphs. Ischaemic heart disease death rates for 1970 and 1975 are not quite comparable to the data for other years. See text for additional explanations.

Figure 6.2 Trends in male and female rates of having a driving licence, cigarette smoking and heavy drinking, USA, 1950–90

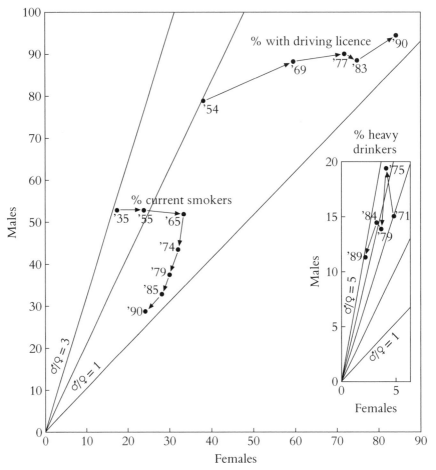

and lung cancer mortality (Burbank 1972; Brown and Kessler 1988; Waldron 1995a). In the early part of the twentieth century, men adopted cigarette smoking earlier and more intensely than women; these trends in smoking account for the early increase in male lung cancer mortality and increasing gender differences in lung cancer mortality during the 1950s (Burbank 1972; Waldron 1991b). In the mid-twentieth century, gender differences in the prevalence of smoking decreased, initially because the prevalence of smoking increased for women and subsequently because the prevalence of smoking decreased more rapidly for men (Figure 6.2; Waldron 1991b). Taking into account the lag of approximately two to three decades between cigarette smoke exposure and lung cancer mortality, the trends in smoking can account for recent increases in female lung cancer mortality and decreases in sex mortality ratios for lung cancer (Figures 6.1 and 6.2; Waldron 1995a). More detailed analyses, which take account of cohort differences and changes in amount of tar consumed per smoker, have shown close relationships between trends in smoking and trends in male and female lung cancer mortality (Lopez 1983; Brown and Kessler 1988). Thus, trends in cigarette smoking have been the primary cause of trends in gender differences in lung cancer mortality. Additional factors which may have played a role include trends in exposures to occupational carcinogens (such as asbestos) and possibly a greater female vulnerability to the carcinogens in cigarette smoke (Waldron 1991a; Zang and Wynder 1996).

Trends in gender differences in cigarette smoking were influenced by trends in gender differences in smoking adoption and, to a lesser extent, by trends in gender differences in smoking cessation (Waldron 1991b). In the early twentieth century, social disapproval of women's smoking was a major cause of women's low rates of smoking adoption. During the mid-twentieth century increasing social acceptance of women's smoking appears to have been a major cause of increased smoking adoption by women. During the 1960s, rates of quitting cigarette smoking were higher for men than for women, probably because, during this early period, the publicity concerning the health damaging effects of smoking had greater relevance for men than for women. More information was available concerning the health risks of smoking for men, and men may have been more responsive to anti-smoking messages since they were more likely to have known someone of their own sex whose health had been adversely affected by smoking. In conclusion, trends in gender differences in smoking appear to have been influenced by trends in social acceptance of women's smoking and men's greater responsiveness to public health campaigns against smoking during the 1960s, as well as several other factors (Waldron 1991b).

International data indicate many similarities between trends in lung cancer mortality in the USA and trends in other Anglophone and western European countries (data from Zarate 1994 and Levi et al. 1996; see also Lopez 1983; Waldron 1993). During the period from 1955 to 1990, lung cancer mortality generally increased, and sex mortality ratios tended to increase initially and then decrease subsequently. However, the timing and magnitude of these trends varied in different countries. Trends in other Anglophone countries tended to be the most similar to the trends in the USA. The major cause of these trends appears to have been trends in male and female smoking habits (Waldron 1993; Koskinen et al. 1994–5; Trovato and Lalu 1998).

Ischaemic heart disease

Ischaemic heart disease is also called coronary heart disease, and a major component of ischaemic heart disease is myocardial infarctions (commonly called heart attacks). In the USA, ischaemic heart disease mortality increased during the 1950s and 1960s, and then decreased substantially during the 1970s and 1980s (Figure 6.1). By 1990, ischaemic heart disease death rates were approximately 40 per cent lower than in 1950.

Males and females showed generally similar proportionate changes in ischaemic heart disease mortality (Figure 6.1). Consequently, sex mortality ratios for ischaemic heart disease were relatively stable, despite large changes in ischaemic heart disease death rates. Unfortunately, changes in the coding of ischaemic heart disease resulted in underestimates of the sex mortality ratios for 1968–78, relative to the other years studied; consequently, trends in sex mortality ratios can be reliably estimated only within each of the three periods with constant or nearly constant coding of ischaemic heart disease deaths. From 1950 to the mid-1960s, the proportionate increase in ischaemic heart disease mortality was somewhat larger for males, so the sex mortality ratio increased slightly from 2.09 in 1950 to 2.21 in 1967. From the late 1960s to the late 1970s, the proportionate decrease in ischaemic heart disease mortality was somewhat larger for females, so the sex mortality ratio increased slightly from 2.05 in 1968 to 2.13 in 1978. From the mid-1970s on, the proportionate decrease in ischaemic heart disease mortality was somewhat larger for males, so the sex mortality ratio decreased slightly from 2.19 in 1979 to 2.05 in 1990. Thus, there appears to have been a slight tendency to increased sex mortality ratios, followed by a slight tendency to decreased sex mortality ratios. However, changes in sex mortality ratios were relatively small, despite large changes in ischaemic heart disease mortality.

Relatively little is known concerning the causes of the early increase in ischaemic heart disease mortality, primarily because relatively little information is available concerning early trends in the multiple factors which influence ischaemic heart disease mortality. During the mid-twentieth century, it appears that increased cigarette smoking and decreased exercise due to mechanization contributed to the increase in ischaemic heart disease mortality (Lopez 1983; Waldron 1995b). Dietary trends do not appear to have been a substantial cause of the increase in ischaemic heart disease mortality in the USA, since unfavourable trends were roughly counterbalanced by favourable trends, such as decreased consumption of butter and lard (Friend 1967; Waldron 1995b).

With respect to the decrease in ischaemic heart disease mortality from the late 1960s on, substantial evidence indicates that these decreases have been due to both improved medical care of ischaemic heart disease patients and decreases in risk factors such as smoking and serum cholesterol levels (Goldman and Cook 1984; Hunink *et al*. 1997). Improvements in cholesterol levels appear to have been due to improved diet, increased exercise and/or increased use of cholesterol lowering medication (Goldman and Cook 1984; Stephens 1987; Johnson *et al*. 1993; Waldron 1997).

Trend data indicate that both males and females have experienced reduced risk factors and increased survival of ischaemic heart disease patients due to improved medical care (Goldman and Cook 1984; Stephens 1987; McGovern *et al*. 1992, 1996; Hunink *et al*. 1997; Waldron 1997). Gender differences in these trends have been relatively small, and trends which have favoured males have been counterbalanced by trends which have favoured females. This appears to be one reason why there has been relatively little variation in sex mortality ratios for ischaemic heart disease. Another reason for the relative stability of sex mortality ratios for ischaemic heart disease may be that biological sex differences make a major contribution to sex differences in ischaemic heart disease mortality (Waldron 1995b; Reis *et al*. 1997). For example, oestrogen appears to have protective effects such as reduced LDL (low-density lipoprotein) cholesterol levels and direct protective effects in coronary artery walls, testosterone may have harmful effects including reduced HDL (high-density lipoprotein) cholesterol levels, and men's greater propensity to accumulate fat in the upper abdomen increases their risk of ischaemic heart disease. Biological influences on sex differences in ischaemic heart disease, together with generally similar improvements in risk factors and medical care for both sexes, probably account for the persistence of sex mortality ratios slightly above 2.0, even while ischaemic heart disease mortality changed dramatically.

Changes in sex mortality ratios for ischaemic heart disease have been small in magnitude, and this is one reason why it is difficult to identify the causes of these trends. Causal analysis is also hampered by data limitations and by the complexity of the multiple interacting factors which influence ischaemic heart disease mortality risk, with both lagged and contemporaneous effects. Despite these difficulties, it is of interest to investigate possible causes of men's slightly more favourable ischaemic heart disease trends during the 1980s.

National data indicate that, during the 1980s, men had somewhat greater decreases in smoking than women, and men had slightly more favourable trends in blood pressure (Figure 6.2; Waldron 1995a; Dustan 1996; Hunink *et al*. 1997; Waldron 1997). However, women had slightly greater improvements in serum cholesterol, possibly due to greater use of cholesterol lowering drugs (Johnson *et al*. 1993; Hunink *et al*. 1997;

Lemaitre *et al.* 1998). Available evidence suggests that other influences on cholesterol trends did not favour women; improvements in exercise and dietary fat intake appear to have been at least as great for men as for women during the 1980s, and both sexes showed similar increases in obesity (Kuczmarski *et al.* 1994; Waldron 1995a, 1997). In summary, trends in some risk factors and health related behaviours favoured men, but others did not.

Current evidence is inconclusive concerning possible gender differences in benefits due to improvements in medical treatment of ischaemic heart disease. A variety of evidence suggests that men may have benefited more, because male patients arrive for treatment with less delay after initial symptoms, male patients are more likely to receive certain types of treatment, and males experience more beneficial and less harmful effects as a result of certain types of treatment (Waldron 1995b; Gurwitz *et al.* 1997; Reis *et al.* 1997; Chandra *et al.* 1998). However, analyses of trends in survival after hospitalization for acute ischaemic heart disease suggest that men and women experienced similar contributions of improved medical treatment to reductions in ischaemic heart disease mortality (McGovern *et al.* 1992, 1996; Rosamond *et al.* 1998). In summary, the factors which contributed to the decrease in ischaemic heart disease mortality showed small and variable gender differences in trends during the 1980s; however, men's somewhat greater decrease in cigarette smoking rates appears to have been one cause of men's slightly greater decrease in ischaemic heart disease mortality.

International data concerning recent trends in ischaemic heart disease mortality indicate several similarities between the USA and other Anglophone or western European countries (Waldron 1993, 1995b; La Vecchia *et al.* 1998). During the 1950s and 1960s, ischaemic heart disease mortality generally increased for men, and sex mortality ratios increased. During the 1970s and 1980s, ischaemic heart disease mortality decreased for both men and women in most Anglophone and western European countries. During the 1970s, females tended to have slightly more favourable trends, so sex mortality ratios tended to increase. In contrast, during the 1980s, males generally had as large or slightly larger proportionate decreases in ischaemic heart disease mortality, so sex mortality ratios were generally stable or decreased slightly.

Detailed analyses of the decreases in ischaemic heart disease mortality during the 1970s and 1980s in two provinces in Finland show many similarities to the patterns observed in the USA (Vartiainen *et al.* 1994; Salomaa *et al.* 1996). The proportionate decrease in ischaemic heart disease mortality was generally similar for men and women. Improved medical treatment of ischaemic heart disease patients appears to have benefited men and women similarly. Another reason for the similar decreases in men's and women's ischaemic heart disease mortality was that the decrease in smoking for men was counterbalanced by greater decreases in serum cholesterol and blood pressure for women. In conclusion, in western European and Anglophone countries, as in the USA, recent trends in ischaemic heart disease mortality have been generally similar for men and women.

Motor vehicle accidents

Motor vehicle accidents mortality in the USA decreased during the 1950s, 1970s and 1980s, but increased during the 1960s (Figure 6.3). The 1960s increase in motor vehicle accidents mortality appears to have been due primarily to increased exposure; vehicle miles travelled increased substantially, with relatively little change in risk of death per mile travelled (Baker *et al.* 1992). During the 1970s and 1980s, vehicle miles travelled continued to increase, but fatality risk per mile travelled decreased substantially, so motor vehicle accidents mortality decreased. The causes of the decrease in fatality risk per mile travelled included improved safety standards for passenger cars and highways, increased seatbelt use, and decreased rates of drinking and driving (Lund and Wolfe 1991; Baker *et al.* 1992; Waldron 1995a, 1998a; Robertson 1996).

Trends in motor vehicle accident mortality tended to be more favourable for males than for females, particularly during the late 1950s and during the 1980s (Figure 6.3). Consequently, sex mortality ratios decreased from 3.4 in 1950 to 2.5 in 1990. These results confirm previous analyses which have shown a general tendency to decreasing gender differences in motor vehicle accidents mortality for various intervals from the late 1950s through the early 1990s (Veevers 1982; National Highway Traffic Safety Administration 1994; Waldron 1995a, 1998a).

To investigate the causes of the trends in gender differences in motor vehicle accident mortality, I have used detailed data which are available for 1970–90 (Waldron 1998a). During this period, sex mortality ratios decreased for the component of motor vehicle accident mortality due to deaths of drivers, while passenger fatalities and pedestrian fatalities showed smaller and inconsistent trends in sex mortality ratios. Therefore, my analysis focuses on causes of changing gender differences in driver fatalities.

The sex mortality ratio for driver fatalities decreased from 5.8 in 1970 to 5.0 in 1980, and decreased further to 3.4 in 1990. One major cause of decreasing gender differences in driver fatalities was decreasing gender differences in amount of driving. Sex ratios decreased for the proportion

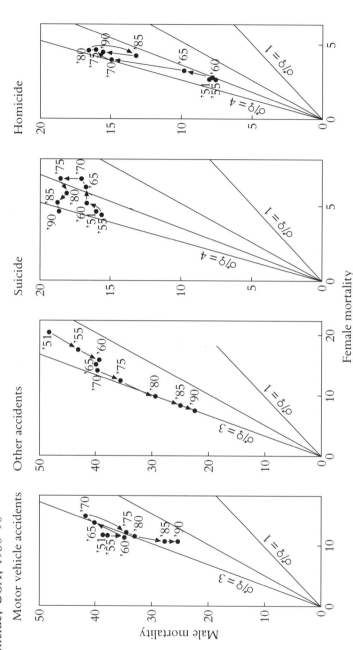

Figure 6.3 Trends in male and female mortality for motor vehicle accidents, other accidents, suicide and homicide, USA, 1950–90

Note: Male and female mortality are shown as age-adjusted death rates per hundred thousand population. Note that scales differ for the different component graphs.

who were licensed drivers and for miles driven per adult, as more women became drivers and women drivers drove more (Figure 6.2; Veevers 1982; National Highway Traffic Safety Administration 1994; Waldron 1995a, 1997, 1998a). Gender differences in driver safety showed mixed trends, depending on the measure and time period considered (Veevers 1982; National Highway Traffic Safety Administration 1994; Waldron 1995a, 1997, 1998a). Sex ratios for driver fatalities per mile driven decreased during the 1970s, but not during the 1980s. It is not known to what extent the 1970s decrease in gender differences in risk of driver fatalities may have been due to decreased gender differences in risky driving habits (for example, speeding) or decreased gender differences in driving in situations with higher fatality risk (for example, night-time driving). Decreasing gender differences have not been observed for several other measures of safety behaviour. With respect to seatbelt use, limited data suggest that during the 1960s and 1970s females were no more likely than males to use seatbelts; during the 1980s females increased their rates of seatbelt use more than males, resulting in an increasing gender difference favouring females (Fhaner and Hane 1973; Helsing and Comstock 1977; Waldron 1997, 1998a). With respect to drinking and driving, inconsistent trends have been observed for gender differences in the proportion of drivers who have elevated blood alcohol levels (Lund and Wolfe 1991; Waldron 1995a, 1998a). In this context, it is of interest that gender differences in the prevalence of heavy drinking have also shown inconsistent trends during the 1970s and 1980s (Figure 6.2; Waldron 1995a, 1997).

In summary, male and female motor vehicle accident mortality increased during the 1960s due to increased miles travelled. Subsequently, motor vehicle accident mortality decreased due to improved safety of cars and highways and improved safety behaviour. Male death rates have tended to decrease proportionately more than female death rates, so sex mortality ratios for motor vehicle accident mortality have tended to decrease. Decreasing gender differences in motor vehicle accident mortality have been due to decreasing gender differences in amount of driving and possibly also decreasing gender differences in driver safety. However, gender differences have not decreased for some types of safety behaviour, such as seatbelt use.

Data for other Anglophone and western European countries indicate that, during 1955–89, trends were generally similar to those observed in the USA. In most countries, motor vehicle accidents mortality showed an early increase, followed by a subsequent decrease, and sex mortality ratios for motor vehicle accidents generally decreased (data from Zarate 1994; Waldron 1993, 1998a). No evidence was found to evaluate whether these similar trends were due to similar causes.

Other accidents

The other accidents category constitutes a diverse group of unintentional injuries due to falls, drownings, fires, poisoning, firearms and other causes, excluding motor vehicle accidents. During the 1950–90 study period, other accidents mortality decreased for both males and females, due in large part to improved medical care and improved safety regulations and safety features, such as better workplace safety and safer domestic gas (Figure 6.3; Baker *et al.* 1984, 1992; Waldron 1998a). The biggest gender difference in trends occurred during the 1960s, when other accidents mortality decreased for females, but not for males (Figure 6.3). In addition, the proportionate decrease in other accidents mortality tended to be greater for females than for males during the 1950s and 1970s. Consequently, sex mortality ratios for other accidents increased from 2.3 in 1950 to 3.0 in 1990.

Trends in gender differences have varied for different types of other accidents. Data for 1960 to 1990 indicate the following trends (Waldron 1998a). For accidental falls, sex mortality ratios increased during the earlier decades, because females experienced proportionately greater decreases in accidental falls mortality. These trends were observed primarily among the elderly, and it appears that improved medical care has been an important cause of the substantial decrease in accidental falls mortality among the elderly people. It has been suggested that improved medical care reduced accidental falls mortality more for women than for men, because men more often fall from a significant height and men's more serious falls may be more immediately lethal (Baker *et al.* 1984, 1992).

For accidental poisonings, sex mortality ratios increased during the 1960s and especially during the 1980s, due to greater increases in accidental poisonings mortality for males. During the 1980s, much of the increase in fatal accidental poisonings was due to increased heroin and cocaine poisonings; these drug overdose fatalities are much more common among males, and consequently the increase in heroin and cocaine poisonings was a major cause of the increase in sex mortality ratios for accidental poisonings (Waldron 1998a).

In contrast, sex mortality ratios for workplace accidents decreased during the 1960s and 1970s, due to greater decreases in fatal workplace accidents for males. During the 1960s, the sex ratio for the proportion of adults employed in blue collar occupations decreased, and this presumably was one important reason why the sex ratio for fatal workplace accidents decreased (Waldron 1998a).

Sex mortality ratios for drownings decreased, due to greater decreases in accidental drownings for males. Sex mortality ratios for firearm accidents decreased initially, but during the 1980s the sex mortality ratio for firearm accidents increased substantially, due to a larger proportionate decrease in firearm accidents mortality for females. The causes of these trends are unclear (Waldron 1998a).

In summary, improved safety regulations and medical care have contributed to decreases in other accidents mortality in the USA. Trends in sex mortality ratios have varied for different types of accidents, reflecting the diverse causal factors which have influenced mortality trends for different types of accidents. Sex mortality ratios for accidental poisonings increased during the 1980s, due primarily to the disproportionate impact of increased illicit drug use on male accidental poisonings mortality. In contrast, sex mortality ratios for workplace accidents decreased during earlier decades, due in part to decreasing gender differences in blue collar employment.

International data show widespread decreases in other accidents mortality, but varied trends in sex mortality ratios in different countries (data from Zarate 1994; Waldron 1998a). Several Anglophone countries experienced increasing sex mortality ratios for other accidents, similar to the USA.

Suicide

Males and females have had very different trends in suicide mortality during the 1950–90 study period in the USA (Figure 6.3). During the 1960s, male suicide rates were relatively stable, while female suicide rates increased; consequently, gender differences in suicide decreased. In contrast, during the 1970s and 1980s, male suicide rates increased, while female suicide rates decreased; consequently, gender differences in suicide increased. Thus, the sex mortality ratio for suicide decreased from 3.3 in 1960 to 2.5 in 1970, and then increased to 4.2 in 1990. Previous analyses have also shown that gender differences in suicide reached a minimum around 1970, due primarily to maximum female suicide rates at about that time (Austin *et al.* 1992; Waldron 1998b). The causes of these trends are unclear, but it appears likely that multiple causal factors have played a role.

One hypothesis proposes that economic trends contributed to the changing gender differences in suicide (Waldron 1995a, 1998b). Several lines of evidence indicate that the economic position of women relative to men worsened during the 1960s, and this may have contributed to the increase in women's suicide and decrease in gender differences in suicide during the 1960s. During the 1970s and 1980s, trends in the economic position of women relative to men differed depending on the economic indicator considered, so it is difficult to evaluate the contribution of economic trends to the trends in gender differences in suicide for this period (Bianchi 1995; Waldron 1995a, 1998b).

A second hypothesis proposes that, during the 1960s and early 1970s, rapid changes in women's roles and attitudes toward women's roles contributed to increased anomie (a lack of generally agreed upon norms and values); increasing anomie is hypothesized to have contributed to increasing female suicide rates during the 1960s, followed by decreasing anomie and decreasing female suicide during subsequent decades (Austin *et al.* 1992). Limited data provide some support for the hypothesized contribution of changes in attitudes toward women's roles. It appears that attitude change was relatively rapid during the early 1970s, when female suicide rates were highest (Mason *et al.* 1976; Spitze and Huber 1980; Cherlin and Walters 1981; Waldron 1998b). There is less support for the hypothesized contribution of increases in women's employment, since women's labour force participation rates continued to increase rapidly during the later period when women's suicide rates were decreasing.

A third hypothesis proposes that trends in gender differences in suicide were influenced by trends in marriage and divorce. Specifically, being married reduces suicide more for men than for women, so decreases in the proportion married would be expected to contribute to increases in the male excess for suicide (National Center for Health Statistics 1967; Smith *et al.* 1988; Waldron 1998b). Previous analyses indicate that recent decreases in the proportion married and increases in the proportions never married and divorced probably account for a small part of the increase in gender differences in suicide during the 1970s and 1980s (Austin *et al.* 1992; Waldron 1995a). However, for the earlier period, the predicted effect of trends in marital status is opposite to the observed changes in gender differences in suicide (Austin *et al.* 1992).

In summary, gender differences in suicide mortality reached a minimum around 1970, due to maximum female suicide rates during that period. The causes of these trends are uncertain. During the earlier period, a growing economic disadvantage for women relative to men and rapid changes in attitudes towards women's roles may have contributed to increasing female suicide rates and decreasing gender differences in suicide. During subsequent decades, decreases in the proportion married probably contributed to increasing suicide for men and increasing gender differences in suicide. Other causal factors have probably also contributed to the trends in gender differences in suicide (Austin *et al.* 1992; Waldron 1998b).

International data show diverse trends in suicide mortality and sex mortality ratios during the 1950–90 study period (data from Zarate 1994; Pampel 1998; Waldron 1998b). In the other Anglophone countries, as in the USA, sex mortality ratios for suicide generally reached a minimum sometime between the late 1960s and the late 1970s.

Homicide

Homicide mortality in the USA has increased substantially, although not consistently, during the 1950–90 study period (Figure 6.3). Increases in homicide mortality have generally been proportionately larger for males than for females, so sex mortality ratios have tended to increase when homicide rates increased (Figure 6.3; Waldron 1998b). For example, during the late 1960s homicide death rates and sex mortality ratios both increased. Conversely, when homicide death rates briefly decreased during the early 1980s, sex mortality ratios also decreased.

Gender differences in committing homicide have been assessed for the period 1960–90, by calculating the sex ratio for rates of arrest as homicide perpetrators (Waldron 1998b). From 1960 to 1990, the sex ratio for committing homicide increased dramatically, from 4.9 to 9.0. During the same period, the sex ratio for homicide mortality increased from 3.0 to 3.9. Thus, in recent decades, gender differences in committing homicide have increased more than gender differences in homicide mortality.

In order to understand these trends, it is useful to distinguish between same-sex and opposite-sex homicides (Waldron 1998b). In the USA, over 90 per cent of same-sex homicides involve males killing males; same-sex homicides are responsible for approximately three-quarters of male homicide deaths, but only about one-tenth of female homicide deaths. During the 1960s, it appears that male–male homicides increased more rapidly than other types of homicides, and the increase in male–male homicides appears to have been the primary cause of the increase in male homicide deaths and perpetrators (Block and Zimring 1973; Rushforth *et al.* 1977; Waldron 1998b). A major component of the increase in male–male homicides was an increase in homicides committed during the course of a robbery or other felony. This trend may have been due in part to increased drug use and drug trafficking. Thus, increased drug-related crime may have been one important cause of increased rates of male homicide victims and perpetrators during the 1960s.

Among opposite-sex homicides, approximately 40 per cent involve victims killed by a spouse and almost 20 per cent involve victims killed by a boyfriend or girlfriend (Waldron 1998b). Rates of opposite sex homicides and rates of spousal homicides have decreased since the late 1970s (Mercy and Saltzman 1989; Browne and Williams 1993; Waldron 1998b). The rate of females killing males has decreased more than the rate of males killing females; similarly, the rate of wives killing husbands has decreased more than the rate of husbands killing wives. This difference appears to relate to the differing motives for murders by wives or husbands. Wives' murders of husbands are often motivated by self-defence or attempts to end physical abuse by their husbands. The decrease in wives killing husbands appears to have been related to increased resources for battered women and increased divorce rates, so that women were more able to escape abusive marriages and apparently as a result were less likely to murder their husbands (Mercy and Saltzman 1989; Browne and Williams 1993; Waldron 1998b). Paradoxically, increased opportunities for battered women to leave their husbands may have had less effect on rates of husbands killing wives, since husbands who murder wives are often motivated by a wife's attempt to leave the relationship, and marital separation is associated with elevated risk of a wife being killed by her husband (Wilson and Daly 1993). In summary, since the late 1970s, increased resources for battered women and increased divorce rates appear to have been important causes of decreased rates of women killing men, while there was less decrease in men killing women. The greater decrease in women killing men would tend to contribute to decreasing proportions of females among homicide perpetrators, but increasing proportions of females among homicide victims. This explains why there were different trends in gender differences for homicide perpetrators and homicide victims, with a greater increase in the male excess for homicide perpetrators.

In summary, trends in gender differences in homicide mortality and homicidal behaviour appear to have been influenced by a variety of social trends, including increased drug-related crime and increased resources for battered women. It is unclear to what extent the trends observed in the USA may generalize to other countries. International data show a general tendency to increasing homicide mortality (data from Zarate 1994; Waldron 1998b). Trends in sex mortality ratios for homicide have varied in different western countries, but in most Anglophone countries sex mortality ratios for homicide have tended to increase when homicide mortality increased, similar to the pattern in the USA.

Total mortality

Total mortality generally decreased for females throughout the study period, but male mortality showed less consistent trends (Figure 6.1). During the early decades, total mortality decreased proportionately more for females than for males, so the sex mortality ratio increased from 1.45 in 1950 to 1.80 in the late 1970s. In contrast, during the 1980s, total mortality decreased proportionately more for males, so the sex mortality ratio decreased slightly from 1.80 in 1980 to 1.74 in 1990. Previous analyses have shown similar trends for sex differences in life expectancy, which increased to a maximum in the late 1970s, and then decreased through 1990 (National Center for Health Statistics 1978–95).

Previous research indicates that, during the 1950s and 1960s, increasing gender differences in total mortality were due to more favourable mortality trends for females for multiple causes of death (Enterline 1961; Gee and Veevers 1983; United Nations 1988; Knudsen and McNown 1993). Females benefited more from decreasing mortality for uterine cancer, maternal mortality, strokes and hypertensive heart disease. Males were affected more by increasing mortality for ischaemic heart disease and lung cancer, and these causes of death were major contributors to the increasing sex ratios for total mortality and the increasing sex differences in life expectancy.

During the 1980s, decreasing mortality for ischaemic heart disease and accidents were major causes of decreasing total mortality for both males and females (Figures 6.1 and 6.3; Waldron 1995a). During this period, ischaemic heart disease mortality and motor vehicle accidents mortality decreased proportionately more for males, and these trends contributed to the modest decrease in sex mortality ratios for total mortality. In addition, lung cancer and chronic obstructive pulmonary disease increased for females, but not for males, and this was the other major reason why sex mortality ratios for total mortality decreased during the 1980s (Waldron 1995a).

International data show generally similar trends to those observed in the USA. For developed countries from the early 1950s to the mid-1970s, proportionate decreases in total mortality were larger and more consistent for females than for males, so sex mortality ratios increased (United Nations 1982). During this period, increasing male disadvantages for ischaemic heart disease and lung cancer were major contributors to the increase in sex mortality ratios for total mortality and the increase in sex differences in life expectancy (United Nations 1982, 1988; Lopez 1983). In contrast, during the 1980s, trends in gender differences in mortality varied in different countries. Decreasing sex mortality ratios and decreasing sex differences in life expectancy were observed primarily in Anglophone and northern European countries. Major causes of the decreasing gender differences in total mortality included decreasing gender differences for lung cancer mortality and, in some countries, decreasing gender differences for ischaemic heart disease mortality (Waldron 1993; Koskinen *et al.* 1994–5; Trovato and Lalu 1998).

Conclusion

The evidence presented in this chapter demonstrates that trends in death rates and trends in sex mortality ratios have been highly variable for different causes of death and different time periods during the 1950–90 study period in the USA. These varied mortality trends reflect the effects of multiple, diverse causal factors. To clarify the general patterns which can be observed in these varied trends and causal relationships, the following paragraphs synthesize the evidence related to each of the descriptive questions and causal hypotheses presented in the introduction to the chapter.

The first descriptive question was: have death rates for each cause of death decreased or increased? Death rates are generally expected to decrease over time, due to improvements in medical care, public health and safety, and standard of living. This expectation is confirmed by some, but not all, of the mortality data presented. Total mortality and other accidents mortality generally decreased, and motor vehicle accidents mortality and ischaemic heart disease mortality decreased from about 1970 on. These decreases in mortality were due to multiple causes, including improvements in medical care, improvements in safety features in workplace environments, roads and cars, and individual changes in behaviour, such as decreased smoking and increased seatbelt use. In contrast, mortality increased for many causes of death during at least part of the time period studied. Considering the whole time period from 1950 to 1990, death rates increased for lung cancer, homicide and, for males only, suicide. These increases in mortality were due to the lagged effects of earlier increases in cigarette smoking and other changes in behaviour and social and economic conditions. Thus, our results are in accord with previous findings which indicate that, due to improving conditions, death rates generally decrease, but stable or increasing death rates are observed under some circumstances (Preston 1976; United Nations 1982; Waldron 1993).

With respect to gender differences in mortality trends and consequent trends in sex mortality ratios, different causes of death showed different patterns (Figures 6.1 and 6.3; Table 6.1). For ischaemic heart disease, men and women experienced similar proportionate changes in death rates, so sex mortality ratios were relatively stable despite large changes in death rates. This result is in accord with the hypothesis that many of the factors which influence mortality trends have similar effects on males and females. Men and women derived generally similar benefits from the improvements in medical care and risk factors which contributed to recent decreases in ischaemic heart disease mortality. Also, trends which favoured men were roughly counterbalanced by trends which favoured women. In contrast, for the other causes of death analysed, trends in important causal factors have influenced one sex more than the other, so males and females experienced different mortality trends and sex mortality ratios changed during at least part of the period studied. Considering the entire period from 1950 to 1990, sex mortality ratios tended to

Table 6.1   Summary of trends in sex ratios for mortality and health related behaviour, USA, 1950–90

Overall trend in sex ratios	Causes of death	Behaviours
Decrease	Motor vehicle accidents Accidental drownings	Having a driving licence Cigarette smoking Blue-collar employment
Tendency to decrease, but inconsistent or weak	Lung cancer Workplace accidents	
Inconsistent and/or weak	Ischaemic heart disease Firearm accidents Homicide Suicide	Exercise Consumption of atherogenic fats Heavy drinking Driving with high blood alcohol (per mile driven)
Tendency to increase, but inconsistent or weak	Accidental poisonings Accidental falls Total mortality	
Increase		Committing homicide

Note: Distinctions between adjacent trend categories are imprecise. Both mortality and behavioural trends are based on national data. Data are for 1950–90, except that data for specific types of non-motor vehicle accidents and committing homicide are for 1960–90, and data for exercise, heavy drinking and driving with high blood alcohol are for 1970–90. See the figures and text for additional trend data.

decrease for lung cancer, motor vehicle accidents, workplace accidents and accidental drownings (Table 6.1). Factors which contributed to these mortality trends include decreasing gender differences in smoking, driving and blue-collar employment. In contrast, sex mortality ratios tended to increase for accidental falls and accidental poisonings. For suicide, homicide and firearm accidents, sex mortality ratios showed both substantial increases and substantial decreases.

With regard to the causes of changing gender differences in mortality, the first hypothesis proposed that trends in cigarette smoking have been a major cause of changing gender differences in mortality. Evidence from this and previous studies supports this hypothesis (Lopez 1983; United Nations 1988; Koskinen *et al.* 1994–5; Waldron 1995a). Initial increases and subsequent decreases in gender differences in smoking have contributed to initial increases and subsequent decreases in gender differences for lung cancer and respiratory diseases and, to a limited extent, for ischaemic heart disease and total mortality.

The second hypothesis proposed that increases in women's labour force participation during the 1950–90 study period have contributed to increases in female mortality and decreases in gender differences in mortality. In accord with this hypothesis, the present analysis indicates that decreasing gender differences in blue-collar employment contributed to decreasing sex mortality ratios for workplace accidents during the first half of the period studied. However, this was a relatively minor effect quantitatively, and, in general, little evidence was found for effects of women's employment on mortality trends. This is in agreement with previous results which indicate that trends in women's labour force participation have had little direct effect on trends in gender differences in health-related behaviour or mortality (Waldron 1993, 1995a, 1997).

The Women's Emancipation Hypothesis proposes that, due to changing gender roles and the concomitant liberalization of norms concerning women's behaviour, gender differences in health related behaviour have decreased, resulting in decreasing gender differences in mortality. The predicted decreases in gender differences were observed for some types of health related behaviour, but not for others (Table 6.1). Specifically, gender differences have decreased for smoking, driving and blue-collar employment, as rates of these behaviours increased more for females and/or decreased more for males. However, gender differences have shown weak and inconsistent trends for exercise, dietary fat intake, heavy drinking, and the propensity to drink and drive. Furthermore, available evidence suggests an increasing male disadvantage for other behaviours such as seatbelt use and committing homicide. In summary, the results of this and previous analyses indicate that recent trends toward decreasing differences in male and female roles have not resulted in a general trend toward decreasing gender differences in health related behaviour (Waldron 1995a, 1997). Rather, gender differences in different types of health related behaviour have shown diverse trends during the 1950–90 study period.

The Gender Roles Modernization Hypothesis proposes that trends in gender differences in behaviour have been influenced by fundamental aspects of traditional gender roles, interacting with contemporary conditions. One prediction is that women are more likely to adopt certain types of behaviour, namely, those which can be viewed as fulfilling fundamental responsibilities of traditional female roles in the modern world (Waldron 1997). For example, increasing proportions of women have driving licences and jobs, and both driving and employment provide ways in which women can meet their families' needs in the contemporary context. In addition, decreasing gender differences in cigarette smoking appear to have been due in part to increasing female use of smoking for weight control, which is compatible with the traditional emphasis on appearance for females (Waldron 1991b). In contrast, heavy drinking is likely to be incompatible with traditional female responsibilities for childcare and sexual restraint; correspondingly, gender differences in heavy drinking remain large. These observations suggest that fundamental aspects of traditional gender roles continue to influence changing gender differences in health related behaviour. It appears that female rates have increased and gender differences have decreased for behaviours which can help a woman to meet female responsibilities for family care and feminine beauty under contemporary conditions, but not for behaviours which are incompatible with traditional female responsibilities for family care and sexual restraint.

Other aspects of the Gender Roles Modernization Hypothesis generally were not supported by the evidence reviewed. For example, this hypothesis predicted that women would respond more to public health campaigns because the female gender role places greater emphasis on preserving health. As predicted, females have increased their use of seatbelts more than males. However, females have not shown better trends than males for several other behaviours which have been promoted in recent public health campaigns. For example, available evidence indicates that improvements in dietary fat intake have not been greater for women than for men. No consistent trends were observed in gender differences in the propensity to drink and drive. Furthermore, since widespread publicity about the health risks of smoking began in the 1960s, men have decreased their smoking rates more than women have. The trends in smoking illustrate the importance of specific factors which may influence gender differences in the response to public health campaigns. For example, it appears that during the 1960s men may have been more responsive to anti-smoking messages, since more information was available concerning the health risks of smoking for men, and men were more likely to have known someone of their own sex whose health had been adversely affected by smoking (Waldron 1991b). In summary, it appears that women have not been consistently more responsive to public health campaigns. This result is congruent with previous findings which indicate that gender differences in explicit health concerns appear to make only limited contributions to gender differences in health related behaviour (Waldron 1991b, 1997). Similarly, very little evidence was found for the increased gender differences in risky behaviour which were predicted to result from the increased proportion of men who do not live with children; this is compatible with previous evidence indicating only small and inconsistent effects of parental status on health related behaviour (Umberson 1987; Waldron and Lye 1989).

In summary, in accord with the Gender Roles Modernization Hypothesis, some aspects of traditional gender roles appear to continue to influence trends in gender differences in behaviour. For example, it appears that women have been more likely to adopt behaviours which can contribute to care of the family in the modern context, and women have been less likely to adopt behaviours which are perceived as incompatible with women's responsibility for family care. However, multiple additional factors have also influenced trends in gender differences in behaviour. In future research, it will be of interest to continue to evaluate possible causes of trends in gender differences in health related behaviour, including varied aspects of changes in gender roles, changes in marital status and education, and varied additional factors suggested by this and previous analyses (Waldron 1991b, 1997).

Trends in gender differences in mortality have been influenced by a variety of factors in addition to trends in gender differences in behaviour. For example, during the 1950s and 1960s, improvements in medical care contributed to decreases in maternal mortality and uterine cancer, and these trends in turn contributed to decreasing total mortality for women and increasing gender differences in total mortality (Enterline 1961; Gee and Veevers 1983). It is unclear whether advances in medical treatment have differentially benefited either sex in more recent decades. Other types of environmental effects on trends in gender differences in mortality have been proposed in this and previous analyses (Preston 1976; Lopez 1983; Waldron 1995a, 1995b, 1998a, 1998b).

One interesting question concerns the extent to which the trends observed for the USA during the 1950–90 study period generalize to other Anglophone and western European countries. The evidence reviewed indicates that these countries showed generally similar trends in death rates and sex mortality ratios for some causes of death (ischaemic heart disease and motor vehicle accidents) and for total mortality. However, for other causes of death (lung cancer and suicide), trends were generally similar in the USA and other Anglophone countries, but differed in various western European countries. The limited available evidence suggests that similar mortality trends in different Anglophone and western European countries shared generally similar causes, although there has been significant international variation in the timing and magnitude of certain trends (United Nations 1988; Waldron 1993, 1995b; Koskinen *et al.* 1994–5). In future research, it will be of interest to investigate the cultural factors or other causes which may account for the greater similarity in trends among the Anglophone countries.

In conclusion, gender differences in mortality have shown diverse trends for different causes of death and different time periods during the 1950–90 study period in the USA. Decreasing gender differences in lung cancer, motor vehicle accidents and workplace accidents mortality appear to have been due in large part to decreasing gender differences in smoking, driving and blue-collar employment. However, other types of mortality and health related behaviour have shown increasing gender differences or inconsistent or weak trends in gender differences. These varied trends reflect the multiple, diverse factors which have influenced trends in gender differences in mortality and health related behaviour.

Acknowledgements

It is a pleasure to acknowledge the invaluable assistance of Kianda Addo and Tso Chen in obtaining and analysing the data presented in this chapter. I thank Jessie Eyer for her help in preparing the bibliography and Katie Eyer and Robert Pollak for helpful comments on an earlier draft.

References

Austin, R. L., Bologna, M. and Dodge, H. H. (1992) Sex-role change, anomie and female suicide: a test of alternative Durkheimian explanations, *Suicide and Life-Threatening Behavior*, 22(2): 197–225.

Baker, S. P., O'Neill, B. and Karpf, R. (1984) *The Injury Fact Book*. Lexington, MA: Lexington Press.

Baker, S., O'Neil, B., Ginsburg, M. and Li, G. (1992) *The Injury Fact Book*, 2nd edn. New York: Oxford University Press.

Bianchi, S. M. (1995) Changing economic roles of women and men, in R. Farley (ed.) *State of the Union, America in the 1990s, Volume 1*. New York: Russell Sage Foundation.

Block, R. and Zimring, F. E. (1973) Homicide in Chicago, 1965–1970, *Journal of Research in Crime and Delinquency*, 10(1): 1–12.

Brown, C. C. and Kessler, L. G. (1988) Projections of lung cancer mortality in the United States: 1985–2025, *Journal of National Cancer Institute*, 80: 43–51.

Browne, A. and Williams, K. R. (1993) Gender, intimacy, and lethal violence: trends from 1976 through 1987, *Gender and Society*, 7(1): 78–98.

Burbank, F. (1972) U.S. lung cancer death rates begin to rise proportionately more rapidly for females than for males: a dose–response effect?, *Journal of Chronic Diseases*, 25: 473–9.

Chandra, N. C., Ziegelstein, R. C., Rogers, W. J. *et al.* (1998) Observations of the treatment of women in the United States with myocardial infarction, *Archives of Internal Medicine*, 158: 981–8.

Cherlin, A. and Walters, P. B. (1981) Trends in United States men's and women's sex-role attitudes: 1972 to 1978, *American Sociological Review*, 46: 453–60.

Dustan, H. P. (1996) Gender differences in hypertension, *Journal of Human Hypertension*, 10: 337–40.

Enterline, P. E. (1961) Causes of death responsible for recent increases in sex mortality differentials in the United States, *Millbank Memorial Fund Quarterly*, 39: 312–38.

Fhaner, C. and Hane, M. (1973) Seat belts: factors influencing their use, a literature survey, *Accident, Analysis and Prevention*, 5: 27–43.

Friend, B. (1967) Nutrients in United States food supply, *American Journal of Clinical Nutrition*, 20(8): 907–14.

Gee, E. M. and Veevers, J. E. (1983) Accelerating sex differentials in mortality: an analysis of contributing factors, *Social Biology*, 30(1): 76–85.

Goldman, L. and Cook, E. F. (1984) The decline in ischemic heart disease mortality rates, *Annals of Internal Medicine*, 101: 825–36.

Grove, R. D. and Hetzel, A. M. (1968) *Vital Statistics Rates in the United States 1940–1960*. Washington, DC: US Department of Health, Education, and Welfare.

Gurwitz, J. H., McLaughlin, T. J., Willison, D. J. *et al.* (1997) Delayed hospital presentation in patients who have had acute myocardial infarction, *Annals of Internal Medicine*, 126(8): 593–9.

Helsing, K. J. and Comstock, G. W. (1977) What kinds of people do not use seat belts? *American Journal of Public Health*, 67(11): 1043–50.

Hunink, M. G. M., Goldman, L., Tosteson, A. N. A. *et al.* (1997) The recent decline in mortality from coronary heart disease, 1980–1990, *Journal of American Medical Association*, 277(7): 535–42.

Johnson, C. L., Rifkind, B. M., Sempos, C. T. *et al.* (1993) Declining serum total cholesterol levels among US adults, *Journal of American Medical Association*, 269(23): 3002–8.

Knudsen, C. and McNown, R. (1993) Changing causes of death and the sex differential in the USA, *Population Research and Policy Review*, 12: 27–41.

Koskinen, S., Martelin, T., Martikainen, P. and Valkonen, T. (1994–5) Convergence of lifestyles and trends in the sex mortality ratio among the middle-aged in Finland, *Yearbook of Population Research in Finland*, 32: 32–44.

Kuczmarski, R. J., Flegal, K. M., Campbell, S. M. and Johnson, C. L. (1994) Increasing prevalence of overweight among U.S. adults, *Journal of American Medical Association*, 272(3): 205–11.

La Vecchia, C., Levi, F., Lucchini, F. and Negri, E. (1998) Trends in mortality from major diseases in Europe, 1980–1993, *European Journal of Epidemiology*, 14: 1–8.

Lemaitre, R. N., Furberg, C. D., Newman, A. B. *et al.* (1998) Time trends in the use of cholesterol-lowering agents in older adults, *Archives of Internal Medicine*, 158: 1761–8.

Levi, F., La Vecchia, C., Lucchini, F. and Negri, E. (1996) Worldwide trends in cancer mortality in the elderly, 1955–1992, *European Journal of Cancer*, 32A(4): 652–72.

Lopez, A. D. (1983) The sex mortality differential in developed countries, in A. D. Lopez and L. T. Ruzicka (eds) *Sex Differentials in Mortality*. Canberra: Department of Demography, Australian National University.

Lund, A. K. and Wolfe, A. C. (1991) Changes in the incidence of alcohol-impaired driving in the United States, 1973–1986, *Journal of Studies on Alcohol*, 52(4): 293–301.

McGovern, P. G., Folsom, A. R., Sprafka, J. M. *et al.* (1992) Trends in survival of hospitalized myocardial infarction patients between 1970 and 1985, *Circulation*, 85: 172–9.

McGovern, P. G., Pankow, J. S., Shahar, E. *et al.* (1996) Recent trends in acute coronary heart disease, *New England Journal of Medicine*, 334(4 April): 884–90.

Mason, K. O., Czajka, J. and Arber, S. (1976) Change in US women's sex-role attitudes 1964–1974, *American Sociological Review*, 41(4): 573–96.

Mercy, J. A. and Saltzman, L. E. (1989) Fatal violence among spouses in the United States, 1976–85, *American Journal of Public Health*, 79(5): 595–9.

National Center for Health Statistics (1953–94) *Vital Statistics of the United States, 1950–1990; Vol. II, Mortality*. Hyattsville, MD: US Department of Health, Education, and Welfare/US Department of Health and Human Services.

National Center for Health Statistics (1967) Suicide in the United States 1950–1964, *Vital and Health Statistics*, Series 20, no. 5.

National Center for Health Statistics (1973) Mortality trends: age, color, and sex, United States, 1950–69, *Vital and Health Statistics*, series 20, no. 15.

National Center for Health Statistics (1974) Mortality trends for leading causes of death, United States, 1950–69, *Vital and Health Statistics*, series 20, no. 16.

National Center for Health Statistics (1978) *Chartbook for the Conference on the Decline in Coronary Heart Disease Mortality*. Hyattsville, MD: US Department of Health, Education, and Welfare.

National Center for Health Statistics (1978–95) Advance report of final mortality statistics, 1978–1995, *Monthly Vital Statistics Report* 26–43, supplements. Hyattsville, MD: Department of Health and Human Services.

National Center for Health Statistics (1980) Estimates of selected comparability ratios based on dual coding of 1976 death certificates by the Eighth and Ninth Revisions of the International Classification of Diseases, *Monthly Vital Statistics Report* 28(11). Hyattsville, MD: US Department of Health, Education and Welfare.

National Center for Health Statistics (1992) *Health, United States, 1991*. Hyattsville, MD: Public Health Service.

National Center for Health Statistics (1995) *Health, United States, 1994*. Hyattsville, MD: Public Health Service.

National Highway Traffic Safety Administration (1994) *Female Drivers in Fatal Crashes*. Washington, DC: US Department of Transportation.

Pampel, F. C. (1998) National context, social change, and sex differences in suicide rates, *American Sociological Review*, 63: 744–58.

Piani, A. and Schoenborn, C. (1993) Health promotion and disease prevention, United States, 1990. *Vital and Health Statistics*, series 10, no. 185. Hyattsville, MD: US Department of Health and Human Services.

Preston, S. H. (1976) *Mortality Patterns in National Populations*. New York: Academic Press.

Reis, S. E., Zell, K. A. and Holubkov, R. (1997) Women's hearts are different, *Current Problems in Obstetrics, Gynecology and Fertility*, 20(3): 69–92.

Robertson, L. S. (1996) Reducing death on the road: the effects of minimum safety standards, publicized crash tests, seat belts, and alcohol, *American Journal of Public Health*, 86(1): 31–4.

Robinson, J. P. and Godbey, G. (1997) *Time for Life*. University Park, PA: Pennsylvania State University Press.

Rosamond, W. D., Chambless, L. E., Folsom, A. R. *et al.* (1998) Trends in the incidence of myocardial infarction and in mortality due to coronary heart disease, 1987 to 1994, *New England Journal of Medicine*, 339: 861–7.

Rushforth, N. B., Ford, A. B., Hirsch, C. S. and Adelson, L. (1977) Violent death in a Metropolitan county, *New England Journal of Medicine*, 297(10): 531–8.

Salomaa, V., Miettinen, H., Kuulasmaa, K. *et al.* (1996) Decline of coronary heart disease mortality in Finland during 1983 to 1992: roles of incidence, recurrence and case-fatality, *Circulation*, 94(12): 3130–7.

Schoenborn, C. A. (1988) Health promotion and disease prevention: United States, 1985. *Vital and Health Statistics*, series 10, no. 163. Washington, DC: US Government Printing Office.

Smith, J. C., Mercy, J. A. and Conn, J. M. (1988) Marital status and the risk of suicide, *American Journal of Public Health*, 78(1): 78–80.

Spitze, G. and Huber, J. (1980) Changing attitudes towards women's nonfamily roles, *Sociology of Work and Occupations*, 7(3): 317–35.

Stephens, T. (1987) Secular trends in adult physical activity, *Research Quarterly for Exercise and Sport*, 58(2): 94–105.

Stronks, K., van de Mheen, H. D., Looman, C. W. N. and Mackenbach, J. P. (1996) Behavioural and structural factors in the explanation of socio-economic inequalities in health: an empirical analysis, *Sociology of Health and Illness*, 18(5): 653–74.

Trovato, F. and Lalu, N. M. (1998) Contribution of cause-specific mortality to changing sex differences in life expectancy: seven nations case study, *Social Biology*, 45(1–2): 1–20.

Umberson, D. (1987) Family status and health behaviors: social control as a dimension of social integration, *Journal of Health and Social Behavior*, 28(3): 306–19.

United Nations (1982) *Levels and Trends of Mortality since 1950*. New York: United Nations.

United Nations (1988) Sex differentials in life expectancy and mortality in developed countries: an analysis by age groups and causes of death from recent and historical data, *Population Bulletin of the United Nations*, 25: 65–106.

US Department of Health and Human Services (1980) *The Health Consequences of Smoking for Women: A Report of the Surgeon General*. Rockville, MD: US Department of Health and Human Services.

US Department of Transportation (1993) *Nationwide Personal Transportation Survey: 1990 NPTS Databook: Vol. I*. Washington, DC: Federal Highway Administration.

Vartiainen, E., Puska, P., Pekkanen, J., Tuomilehto, J. and Jousilanti, P. (1994) Changes in risk factors explain changes in mortality from ischaemic heart disease in Finland, *British Medical Journal*, 309: 23–7.

Veevers, J. (1982) Women in the driver's seat: trends in sex differences in driving and death, *Population Research and Policy Review*, 1: 1–11.

Waldron, I. (1991a) Effects of labor force participation on sex differences in mortality and morbidity, in M. Frankenhauser, U. Lundberg and M. Chesney (eds) *Women, Work and Health*. New York: Plenum.

Waldron, I. (1991b) Patterns and causes of gender differences in smoking, *Social Science and Medicine*, 32(9): 989–1005.

Waldron, I. (1993) Recent trends in sex mortality ratios for adults in developed countries, *Social Science and Medicine*, 36(4): 451–62.

Waldron, I. (1995a) Contributions of changing gender differences in behavior and social roles to changing gender differences in mortality, in D. Sabo and D. F. Gordon (eds) *Men's Health and Illness*. Thousand Oaks, CA: Sage.

Waldron, I. (1995b) Contributions of biological and behavioural factors to changing sex differences in ischaemic heart disease mortality, in A. Lopez, G. Caselli and T. Valkonen (eds) *Adult Mortality in Developed Countries: From Description to Explanation*. New York: Oxford University Press.

Waldron, I. (1997) Changing gender roles and gender differences in health behavior, in D. S. Gochman (ed.) *Handbook of Health Research I: Personal and Social Determinants*. New York: Plenum.

Waldron, I. (1998a) Trends in gender differences in motor vehicle and other accidents, 1950–1995. In manuscript.

Waldron, I. (1998b) Trends in gender differences in suicide and homicide, 1950–1995. In manuscript.

Waldron, I. and Lye, D. (1989) Family roles and smoking, *American Journal of Preventive Medicine*, 5(3): 136–41.

Wilson, M. and Daly, M. (1993) Spousal homicide risk and estrangement, *Violence and Victims*, 8(1): 3–16.

Zang, E. A. and Wynder, E. L. (1996) Differences in lung cancer risk between men and women: examination of the evidence, *Journal of the National Cancer Institute*, 88(3/4): 183–92.

Zarate, A. O. (1994) *International Mortality Chartbook*. Hyattsville, MD: Public Health Service.

seven

Gender and socio-economic inequalities in mortality in central and eastern Europe

Laurent Chenet

Introduction

The study of gender inequality in mortality provides us with a well known paradoxical observation: women might still be subordinated in most societies but, in more developed countries, they nevertheless live longer than men. However, in the same way that women's subordination is universal but extremely variable (Ortner 1974), the mortality advantage of women over men takes many different forms, even in countries as close culturally and geographically as those of Europe.

As elsewhere, women can expect to live much longer than men in the countries of central and eastern Europe, but the female advantage in mortality is often much greater, in comparison with western European countries. Moreover, there is ample evidence that the enormous societal changes in the countries of central and eastern Europe following the revolutions of the late 1980s and early 1990s have had a greater negative impact on the health of men than on women. This is despite the fact that, intuitively, we might have expected women to have suffered more from these changes than men.

After explaining why women would be expected to experience greater socio-economic challenges during the transition, this chapter aims to provide an overview of sex mortality differentials in central and eastern Europe, describing the Russian situation in more detail. The final section describes the relationship between gender and socio-economic differentials by analysing individual death records from Moscow, the Russian capital city.

Socio-economic impact of social change on women

Because of their former position under communism, there are various reasons why women should have experienced the political and social transition as more traumatic than men. Under communism, female labour force participation was extremely high, especially when compared to western societies. This high employment level was accompanied by fairly generous tenured maternity leaves, family benefits and childcare facilities. This pattern of female employment has been used as a symbol of successful egalitarian socialist societies (Molyneux 1987). However, most of these policies were founded on economic or pro-natalist aims, rather than a desire to attain gender equality. Indeed, if women were fully employed this was often not through their own choice and the 'hidden curriculum' in education was just as powerful as in the west, leading women to work mostly in services and light industry when heavy industry (much praised under proletarian ideology) remained male territory (Nickel 1993). By and large, women were also kept in positions with less power and less financial remuneration than men (Funk 1993).

After the revolution, women's employment patterns made them particularly vulnerable to redundancy. First, women's full employment was associated with communism and therefore was opposed both by those nostalgic for a pre-communist era, and by the proponents of a new capitalist society (Lissyutkina 1993). Second, maternity and family benefits meant that women were a rather costly labour force and thus particularly vulnerable during the process of economic restructuring (Heitlinger 1993; Moghadam 1993). Finally, along with the economic crisis, the budgetary constraints imposed on the central and eastern European countries, either by the World Bank or the EU for example, meant that childcare facilities were closed. This has made it difficult for women to remain employed in countries where part-time work is not available (Heitlinger 1993).

The second threat to women's health during the transition period has been the introduction of restrictions on abortion. Women in eastern Europe have used abortion as a contraceptive method more than in the west. Pushed out of the workforce back into the home, women saw the right to free abortion restricted either by legislative measures, as in Poland, or simply by the introduction of prohibitive fees as in Russia and the Baltic States (Nowicka 1995; Karro *et al.* 1997; Kozakiewicz 1997). Undoubtedly, some women now turn to illegal, unsafe abortion.

Figure 7.1 Female–male difference in life expectancy at birth, Czechoslovak Republic, Hungary, Poland, 1970–95

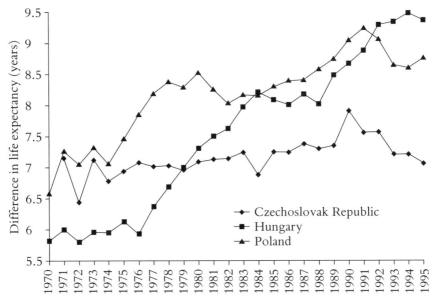

Unfortunately, this may yet continue. Although women had been politically active during the revolutions of central Europe and during the 1992 uprising in the Soviet Union, they now find themselves out of political life, and women's issues are singularly absent from the speeches of their leaders (Eisenstein 1993; Wolchik 1993). Moreover, the budgetary pressure imposed by the EU treaties, along with the reluctance of the private sector to employ women or to provide affordable childcare, means that women with young children will find it hard to secure paid work.

The gender gap in mortality in societies in transition: universal disadvantage for men

Central Europe

In central Europe, life expectancy at birth has been falling for men during the transition, even if only temporarily, in virtually every country. This has not really happened for women for whom life expectancy at birth stagnated until the early 1990s. As a result, the difference in male–female life expectancy increased dramatically during the late 1980s and early 1990s, most strikingly in Hungary as illustrated in Figure 7.1. The

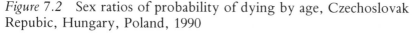

Figure 7.2 Sex ratios of probability of dying by age, Czechoslovak Repubic, Hungary, Poland, 1990

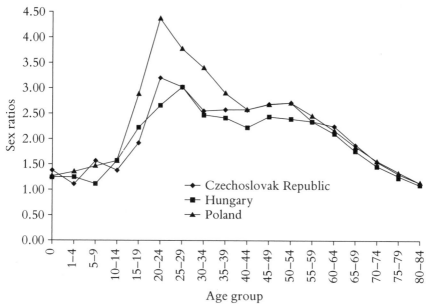

difference in male–female life expectancy at birth reached over nine years in Hungary and Poland and nearly eight years in the (then) Czechoslovak Republic at the beginning of the 1990s. Thereafter, this difference started to decrease again during the stabilization period, except maybe in Hungary where male life expectancy went on decreasing until 1993. The similarities of the curves between the three countries suggest a very similar pattern of mortality in all three countries.

Figure 7.2 shows the ratio of the probability of dying (male/female) by age for Poland, Hungary and the (then) Czechoslovak Republic in 1990, the year following the fall of the Berlin Wall when all central European countries experienced painful economic hardship. Once again the similarities between the three, typically bimodal, curves are striking. Excess male mortality at all ages is apparent, with a peak during young adulthood and a later (but less pronounced) peak around age 50. However, both the difference in life expectancy and in probability of dying are not very different from what can be observed in the EU countries that are also characterized by high male excess mortality, such as France or Finland.

However, examination of these sex ratios of probability of dying by age does not give a clear picture of the contribution of these probabilities to the overall male–female difference in life expectancy. Figure 7.3

Figure 7.3 Contribution to female–male difference in life expectancy (in years) by age group, Czechoslovak Republic, Poland, Hungary, 1990

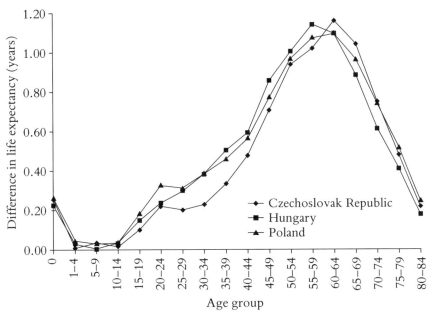

shows the result of a component analysis of the male–female difference in life expectancy at birth by age (for a discussion of the method see Pollard 1982, 1987; for its application to central European countries see Chenet *et al.* 1996; McKee *et al.* 1996). Using this method we can see that the huge difference in life expectancy at birth between men and women is mostly due to excess male mortality between the ages of 40 and 70. Although mortality among young men is higher in the countries of central Europe than it is in the west, it remains sufficiently low at these ages for the extraordinary peaks displayed in Figure 7.2 to have only a small impact on the overall difference in life expectancy, as seen in the west (Vallin 1996).

It is also possible to use the component analysis method to look at the contribution of various causes of deaths to the gender difference in life expectancy at birth. The results for 1990 are given in Table 7.1. Although the pattern is broadly similar in the three countries, there are some striking differences. In Hungary, suicide and liver cirrhosis account for a much higher proportion of the difference between male and female life expectancy. In Poland, accidents and violence (excluding suicide) represent 1.79 years of the 9 years' difference, while diseases of

Table 7.1 Contribution of cause of death to the male–female difference in life expectancy (in years), Czechoslovak Republic, Poland, Hungary, 1990

	Czechoslovak Republic	*Poland*	*Hungary*
Infectious disease	−0.03	−0.12	−0.10
Neoplasm	−1.77	−1.55	−1.73
Ischaemic heart disease	−2.33	−1.71	−1.82
Other cardiovascular	−1.07	−1.84	−1.31
Respiratory disease	−0.47	−0.45	−0.45
Congenital perinatal	−0.23	−0.21	−0.16
Chronic liver cirrhosis	−0.46	−0.14	−0.67
Accidents, violence	−1.16	−1.79	−1.34
Suicide	−0.39	−0.42	−0.74
Other	−0.46	−0.86	−0.50
Total	−8.38	−9.08	−8.83

the circulatory system represent a further 3.55 years. There has been a tendency to look at the countries of central Europe as a rather homogenous group despite important cultural and historical differences. However, because male excess mortality is very much linked to cultural and behavioural factors, such as acceptance of smoking or drunkenness, cultural differences will have an important influence on the pattern of male excess mortality.

The importance of cardiovascular diseases and neoplasms at older ages in explaining the gender gap in mortality is often overlooked in favour of the more newsworthy accidents, violence and suicides that are mostly responsible for excess male mortality observed before the age of 40. However, diseases of the circulatory system present a particular challenge to countries in transition since the fight against degenerative diseases in these countries has yet to begin in earnest. There has been very little concerted action so far to fight tobacco smoking and alcohol consumption in the countries of central Europe. For example, in Hungary where liver cirrhosis is rising with epidemic characteristics (Varvasovszky *et al.* 1997), it is virtually impossible to find anyone taking responsibility for the fight against alcohol consumption (Varvasovszky and McKee 1998). Because men are more likely to smoke or drink excessively than women, they are also more prone to die from these diseases, hence the very important differences in life expectancy at birth. Another aspect of the lack of health policy to fight these diseases is the fact that in the west women have often been the first to heed the messages for a healthier lifestyle, and to take advantage of coherent health promoting measures (Vallin 1988, 1996). It is therefore possible that if such policies are introduced in central European countries, women's life expectancy will initially increase much faster than men's.

Russia

Until the second half of the twentieth century, life expectancy at birth in Russia lagged well behind western European levels. However, after the Second World War progress was so rapid that in 20 years, life expectancy at birth in Russia nearly caught up with that of western Europe. Since the mid-1960s, however, there has been no further convergence of Russian mortality towards western levels. As in central European countries, the earlier success of the fight against infectious agents was followed by a failure to curtail rising cardiovascular and cancer mortality rates. Moreover, deaths from accidents and violence, as well as alcohol related mortality, remained much higher than in western Europe. During the 1980s, Gorbachev's anti-alcohol campaign had an important impact: in 1987 male life expectancy had reached 65 years and female 74, but this advance was short lived (Ryan 1995). Since then, Russians suffered an unprecedented mortality crisis that had reduced life expectancy to 57 years in men and 71 years in women in 1995, resulting in a male–female difference in life expectancy of nearly 14 years.

Accidental and violent deaths, as well as alcohol related mortality, have played a major role in this mortality crisis, with young adults of working ages being most affected (Meslé *et al.* 1994, 1995). Moreover, not only did mortality rates from alcohol related diseases increase sevenfold (and accidents and violence mortality rates fivefold) for adults in their 40s between 1988 and 1994, but there is also evidence that alcohol played a major role in the increase in cardiovascular mortality (Leon *et al.* 1997).

Men and women showed apparently very similar *relative* decreases and increases in overall mortality. However, mortality rates are much higher for men than for women, and life expectancy for men fell by nearly 8 years as opposed to 'only' 3 years for women. It is worth noting that for all causes and for diseases of the circulatory system (the main cause of death for both sexes in Russia), the increase in mortality rates concerned men in slightly younger age groups, and was also slightly greater than for women (Leon *et al.* 1997).

The sex ratios of the probability of dying for 1987 (when male mortality was at its lowest) and 1994 (when it was at its highest) are shown

Figure 7.4 Sex ratios of probability of dying by age, Russia, 1987 and 1994

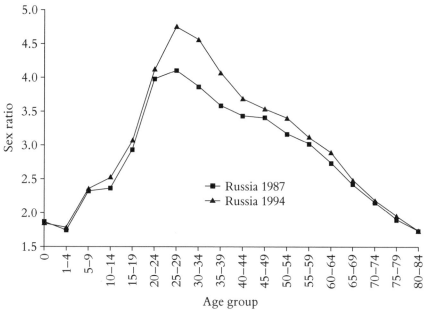

in Figure 7.4. In contrast with the countries of central Europe shown in Figure 7.2, these curves are not bimodal, particularly in 1994. The 1994 curve rises steeply and male mortality is more than 400 per cent higher than female mortality from age 20 to 40. After that, as female mortality rises with age, the differential decreases but remains high.

Thus, the gender difference in life expectancy in Russia can be explained to a much greater extent by male excess mortality at younger ages in comparison with central European countries. Table 7.2 shows the results of a component analysis of the gender difference in life expectancy by cause of death and age group for Russia in 1994. Once again, male mortality is higher for virtually every broad cause of death and every age group (with the exception of breast cancer). However, in contrast with countries of central Europe where the peak of excess male mortality at younger ages made a relatively small contribution to the difference in life expectancy, more than half of the difference in Russia is explained by excess male mortality before the age of 50.

The contribution of accidents and violence to the overall difference in life expectancy is particularly high, much greater than in central Europe, as is the contribution of suicide. Perhaps more striking is the contribution of mortality directly related to alcohol which accounts for

Table 7.2 Contribution to male–female difference in life expectancy (in years), by cause of death and age group, Russia, 1994

	Infectious	Respiratory cancer	Breast cancer	Other neoplasm	Ischaemic heart disease	Other cardiovascular	Respiratory disease	Alcohol related	Suicide	Accidents and violence	Other	Total
0–14	-0.02	0.00	0.00	-0.01	0.00	0.00	-0.05	0.00	-0.01	-0.18	-0.29	-0.57
15–49	-0.25	-0.10	0.09	-0.12	-0.88	-0.50	-0.27	-0.73	-0.87	-3.04	-0.22	-6.89
50–64	-0.12	-0.41	0.09	-0.40	-1.26	-0.57	-0.40	-0.24	-0.19	-0.64	-0.15	-4.29
65+	-0.02	-0.24	0.04	-0.29	-0.71	-0.44	-0.29	-0.02	-0.04	-0.09	-0.07	-2.19
Total	-0.42	-0.75	0.22	-0.82	-2.86	-1.51	-1.02	-0.99	-1.11	-3.95	-0.74	-13.95

one year of the difference in life expectancy between men and women. Other important contributions to the difference come from diseases of the circulatory system: already at ages 40–4, 0.25 year of the difference in life expectancy can be explained by ischaemic heart disease alone. Diseases of the respiratory system and neoplasms also account for a large proportion of the difference but at a later age.

Gender differences and socio-economic inequalities in Moscow

Gender and socio-economic inequalities were not studied under the former Soviet system since they were more or less supposed to have been eradicated. However, recent research has shown that not only were socio-economic inequalities in mortality present in Russia, but also they may be even more important than in the west. Chenet *et al.* (1998a) analysed mortality records for Moscow, the capital city, for the years 1994 and 1995. Because young men had been particularly affected by the mortality crisis, data were originally analysed in order to examine the relationship between socio-economic status and deaths directly related to alcohol, and deaths due to accidents or violence. Here we extend this analysis by also including mortality records for 1993 (to increase statistical power) and by analysing more causes of deaths in order to try and account better for women's deaths during the transition period. Of the 3.2 years of life expectancy lost by Russian women between 1988 and 1994, 1.6 were due to diseases of the circulatory system, 0.84 to accidents and violence and 0.36 to deaths related directly to alcohol. All these causes were therefore analysed.

Data and method

Moscow is not fully representative of Russia, just as London or Copenhagen are not typical of the UK or Denmark (Juel and Sjøl 1995; Charlton 1996). Rather it represents an accentuation of what can be observed elsewhere in Russia. The computerized death certificates analysed contain a wealth of information including education, occupational group, marital status and cause of death. The person who registers the death provides information on the highest educational level attained and the occupation of the deceased. Education is coded into six categories: higher (15–17 years of education); incomplete higher (13–15 years, including those who spent at least 3 years at a university, institute or higher military school); secondary special (11–13 years, including additional training in specific vocational skills for qualified non-manual and manual occupations such as engine driver, cook or nurse); secondary (10–11

Table 7.3 Comparison of Soviet classification of causes of death with ninth revision of the International Classification of Diseases (ICD 9)

Cause of death	Soviet classification	ICD 9 codes
Alcohol related diseases		
Alcohol psychoses	73	291
Alcohol dependence syndrome	75	303
Alcoholic liver cirrhosis	123	571.0–571.3
Diseases of the pancreas	126	577
Accidental poisoning by alcohol	163	860
Accidents and violence (excluding accidental alcohol poisoning)	160–162; 164–175	800–858; 861–999
Cerebrovascular diseases	98–99	430–438
Other diseases of cardiovascular system	84–97; 100–102	390–429; 440–459
All neoplasms	45–67	140–239

years); incomplete secondary (8–10 years); and primary education or less (up to 8 years' education). Given the small numbers in the incomplete higher education category, this category has been merged with higher education. Occupation is coded into non-manual, manual, unemployed not dependent or dependent. 'Unemployed not dependent' concerns people who are not participating in remunerated activities but nevertheless receive an income (from the state for example): students and pensioners would be included in this category. 'Not employed dependent' concerns people who are entirely dependent on their relatives and have no income whatsoever. Marital status (married, never married, widowed, divorced) is taken from the deceased's identification documents that have to be provided when a death is registered. Cause of death is recorded using a unique system of disease classification based on ICD 9 but containing only 175 categories. Correspondence between the Soviet classification and ICD 9 for causes of interest are given in Table 7.3.

In the absence of a proper denominator containing socio-economic characteristics, a proportional mortality analysis was used. This method enables one to estimate whether different subgroups of the population, defined for instance by education, are more or less likely to die from a specific cause of interest than from some other cause of death, taking account of potential confounders such as age. This may be expressed as an odds ratio relative to an arbitrary baseline category. Deaths are therefore analysed within a case-control framework. In Russia, because of the relative stability of mortality from neoplasms over the study period, cancer deaths were used as the control, while the cases were either alcohol related deaths, or accidental or violent deaths (for details of the analysis and a discussion of limitation see McDowall 1983; Chenet *et al.* 1998a). (Because cancer rates are also susceptible to socio-economic differences the controls were originally systematically modified in order to exclude (1) cancer of the lung; (2) cancer of the stomach; (3) cancer of the upper-aero digestive tract (UADT); (4) breast cancer; (5) all of the above, because of their known association with such risk factors as smoking or alcohol consumption. The results were always entirely consistent and all the statistics presented here were obtained with the last series of control (i.e. all cancer minus lung, stomach, UADT, breast).) A logistic regression was then performed (integrating age in the model) generating odds ratios.

Results

The analysis included 125,074 deaths (91,961 male deaths and 33,113 female deaths; sex ratio 2.77) that occurred in Moscow between 1 January 1993 and 31 December 1995 among people aged 20–59 years. Education, occupation and marital status were specified for 95.4 per cent, 89 per cent, and 95.6 per cent of all deaths respectively (Table 7.4).

The results confirm the existence of marked socio-economic differentials in mortality in Moscow; in comparison with men who had reached higher education, men who had completed only secondary education were more than 3 times as likely to die from causes directly related to alcohol, twice as likely to die from accidents or violence, and 1.8 times more likely to die from a disease of the circulatory system (Table 7.4). For women the socio-economic differentials seem to be much stronger (the only exception being the 'other' residual category). In comparison with women who had reached higher education, women who had completed only secondary education were more than 5 times as likely to die from causes directly related to alcohol, twice as likely to die from accidents or violence, and 2.8 times more likely to die from diseases of the circulatory system. For all diseases the difference was even greater for women failing to complete secondary education; for example, these women were over 8 times more likely than women reaching higher education to die of an alcohol related death. The lowest educational category (primary education or less) did not always have the highest odds ratio. However, as secondary education was more or less universal in the former Soviet Union, this group is thought to be highly selected and characterized by physical disability or learning disorders.

Turning to occupational status, male manual workers are twice as likely to die of most causes as men in non-manual occupations, while

Table 7.4 Proportional mortality analysis, Moscow City deaths, age 20–59, by education level, 1993–5 (Odds ratios 95% confidence interval)

Cause of death	Educational status				
	Higher education	Secondary special	Secondary	Secondary incomplete	Primary or less
Men					
Alcohol related mortality	1.00	2.30 (1.99 2.68)	3.28 (2.89 3.72)	4.18 (3.61 4.85)	3.51 (2.60 4.73)
Accidents and violence	1.00	1.59 (1.43 1.76)	2.02 (1.86 2.19)	2.32 (2.09 2.57)	1.81 (1.46 2.25)
Diseases of the circulatory system	1.00	1.5 (1.36 1.65)	1.82 (1.68 1.97)	2.10 (1.9 2.31)	1.85 (1.52 2.26)
Cerebrovascular diseases	1.00	1.67 (1.47 1.88)	1.84 (1.66 2.04)	2.15 (1.91 2.43)	2.36 (1.87 2.97)
Other	1.00	1.88 (1.7 2.08)	2.45 (2.26 2.66)	3.13 (2.83 3.45)	3.21 (2.63 3.91)
Women					
Alcohol related mortality	1.00	2.61 (1.93 3.53)	5.13 (3.92 6.73)	8.54 (6.24 11.70)	5.24 (3.08 8.93)
Accidents and violence	1.00	1.44 (1.25 1.55)	1.96 (1.72 2.23)	2.52 (2.10 3.02)	1.68 (1.18 2.39)
Diseases of the circulatory system	1.00	1.86 (1.66 2.08)	2.79 (2.52 3.09)	3.88 (3.41 4.41)	4.09 (3.32 5.04)
Cerebrovascular diseases	1.00	1.45 (1.26 1.55)	2.08 (1.82 2.36)	2.91 (2.50 3.39)	3.01 (2.36 3.83)
Other	1.00	1.25 (1.14 1.38)	1.59 (1.46 1.74)	2.06 (1.82 2.32)	2.26 (1.85 2.74)

Table 7.5   Proportional mortality analysis, Moscow City deaths, age 20–59, by occupational status, 1993–5 (Odds ratios 95% confidence interval)

Cause of death	Occupational group			
	Non-manual	*Manual*	*Not working, not dependent*	*Not working, dependent*
Men				
Alcohol related mortality	1.00	3.32	0.82	6.24
		2.86 3.85	0.71 0.96	5.23 7.44
Accidents and violence	1.00	2.25	0.46	2.80
		2.03 2.47	0.42 0.51	2.46 3.21
Diseases of the circulatory system	1.00	1.91	0.88	2.69
		1.73 2.11	0.80 0.96	2.36 3.08
Cerebrovascular diseases	1.00	1.84	0.99 ★★	1.86
		1.63 2.08	0.89 1.11	1.58 2.19
Other	1.00	2.51	1.67	3.93
		2.26 2.78	1.52 1.83	3.43 4.51
Women				
Alcohol related mortality	1.00	3.69	0.87 ★★	7.64
		2.80 4.66	0.67 1.15	5.81 10.04
Accidents and violence	1.00	2.18	0.47	2.74
		1.90 2.51	0.42 0.54	2.36 3.19
Diseases of the circulatory system	1.00	2.96	1.14	3.95
		2.54 3.44	1.01 1.30	3.36 4.65
Cerebrovascular diseases	1.00	1.95	0.80	1.84
		1.63 2.32	0.58 0.93	1.51 2.25
Other	1.00	1.83	1.28	2.42
		1.59 2.09	1.15 1.43	2.09 2.80

Notes: ★ significant at the 10% level
★★ not significant

men receiving a state pension are less likely to die from most causes except the residual 'other' category. Unemployed men dependent on relatives for their livelihood are at much higher risk of death from all causes (Table 7.5). For women the pattern is more or less the same.

Marital status presents a more complicated picture. Married men have lower odds ratios than other men for all causes of death and divorced men seem to be most 'at risk' with a probability of dying over twice as high as for married men (with the exception of cerebrovascular disease). For women, the protective effect of marriage is less clear and not statistically significant at the 5 per cent level for diseases of the circulatory system, the biggest killer. Moreover, it seems that the most risky status is being widowed, and not divorced as for men (Table 7.6).

Table 7.6 Proportional mortality analysis, Moscow City deaths, age 20–59, by marital status, 1993–5 (Odds ratios 95% confidence interval)

Cause of death	Marital status			
	Married	Single	Widowed	Divorced
Men				
Alcohol related mortality	1.00	2.19	2.80	3.38
		1.88 2.56	2.15 3.63	3.00 3.82
Accidents and violence	1.00	1.57	2.01	2.57
		1.39 1.77	1.64 2.46	2.31 2.82
Diseases of the circulatory	1.00	1.81	1.88	2.26
system		1.60 2.05	1.56 2.28	2.05 2.49
Cerebrovascular diseases	1.00	1.58	1.93	1.82
		1.36 1.85	1.55 2.40	1.63 2.05
Other	1.00	2.47	2.38	2.72
		2.19 2.78	1.96 2.87	2.47 3.00
Women				
Alcohol related mortality	1.00	1.45	2.66	1.95
		1.13 1.86	2.15 3.30	1.65 2.32
Accidents and violence	1.00	1.33	1.77	1.70
		1.16 1.53	1.54 2.03	1.53 1.88
Diseases of the circulatory	1.00	1.14 ∗	1.61	1.38
system		0.99 1.30	1.44 1.81	1.26 1.52
Cerebrovascular diseases	1.00	1.06 ∗∗	1.55	1.19
		0.89 1.26	1.35 1.77	1.05 1.33
Other	1.00	1.37	1.47	1.36
		1.21 1.55	1.32 1.65	1.24 1.49

Notes: ∗ significant at the 10% level
　　　∗∗ not significant

These analyses show not only that there are socio-economic inequalities in mortality present in Russia but also that these *relative* differentials seem to be greater for women than for men for alcohol related diseases, accidents and violence, cardiovascular and cerebrovascular diseases. However, absolute differentials are greater for men than for women in Russia as in the west (Koskinen and Martelin 1994; Shkolnikov *et al.* 1998).

In a second stage of the analysis, sex was entered directly into the model instead of analysing men and women separately. Thus, for each socio-economic category, the probability of dying from a particular cause is compared between men and women (see Table 7.7). As shown above, the odd ratios of dying from alcohol related diseases, accidents

Table 7.7 Proportional mortality, analysis by Moscow City deaths, age 20–59, men vs women, 1993–5 (Odds ratios 95% confidence interval)

Educational status

Cause of death	Higher education Women	Men		Secondary special Women	Men		Secondary Women	Men		Secondary incomplete Women	Men		Primary or less Women	Men	
Alcohol related mortality	1	6.4	5.03 8.14	1	5.51	4.54 6.70	1	4.00	3.52 4.55	1	3.11	2.54 3.81	1	3.50	2.14 5.72
Accidents and violence	1	4.39	3.97 4.86	1	5.03	4.47 5.66	1	4.68	4.28 5.11	1	4.04	3.50 4.68	1	3.18	2.32 4.37
Diseases of the circulatory system	1	5.25	4.76 5.80	1	4.30	3.05 4.81	1	3.49	3.21 3.80	1	2.74	2.41 3.12	1	2.27	1.73 2.98
Cerebrovascular diseases	1	2.10	1.86 2.37	1	2.45	2.14 2.82	1	1.90	1.72 2.11	1	1.49	1.28 1.74	1	1.53	1.12 2.09
Other	1	1.60	1.46 1.75	1	2.40	2.16 2.68	1	2.48	2.29 2.69	1	2.47	2.17 2.81	1	2.39	1.82 3.14

Occupational group

Cause of death	Non-manual Women	Men		Manual Women	Men		Not working, not dependent Women	Men		Not working, dependent Women	Men	
Alcohol related mortality	1	5.12	3.92 6.68	1	4.27	3.56 5.14	1	3.26	2.80 3.79	1	4.27	3.48 5.23
Accidents and violence	1	4.36	3.81 4.98	1	4.36	3.85 4.94	1	3.07	2.82 3.33	1	4.84	4.08 5.74
Diseases of the circulatory system	1	5.13	4.46 5.89	1	3.49	3.08 3.95	1	3.14	2.93 3.36	1	4.14	3.49 4.90
Cerebrovascular diseases	1	1.89	1.60 2.24	1	1.79	1.55 2.08	1	1.78	1.64 1.94	1	2.06	1.67 2.54
Other	1	1.66	1.46 1.89	1	2.35	2.08 2.66	1	2.12	1.98 2.26	1	2.88	2.44 3.39

Table 7.7 (cont'd)

Cause of death	Marital status							
	Married		Single		Widowed		Divorced	
	Women	Men	Women	Men	Women	Men	Women	Men
Alcohol related mortality	1	4.28	1	6.47	1	4.17	1	6.80
		3.82 4.80		4.96 8.44		3.04 5.73		5.98 7.72
Accidents and violence	1	4.54	1	4.05	1	5.20	1	6.79
		4.24 4.85		4.28 5.95		4.10 6.59		5.98 7.72
Diseases of the circulatory system	1	3.51	1	5.32	1	3.94	1	5.83
		3.31 3.73		4.47 6.32		3.18 4.88		5.17 6.59
Cerebrovascular diseases	1	1.86	1	2.78	1	2.16	1	2.91
		1.73 2.00		2.24 3.46		1.69 2.75		2.51 3.37
Other	1	1.97	1	2.99	1	3.34	1	4.03
		1.86 2.09		2.56 3.50		2.69 4.13		3.58 4.55

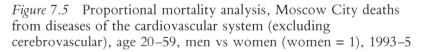

Figure 7.5 Proportional mortality analysis, Moscow City deaths from diseases of the cardiovascular system (excluding cerebrovascular), age 20–59, men vs women (women = 1), 1993–5

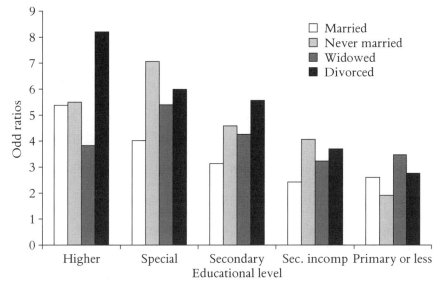

and violence, cardiovascular or cerebrovascular diseases are much greater among those with lower levels of education for both men and women. However, the gap between men and women is actually somewhat greater among the best educated. In other words, the less educated they are, the more equal men and women are!

Koskinen and Martelin (1994) pointed out that marital status had a huge mitigating effect on sex differentials in mortality, with differences between married men and women being smaller than the differences between men and women in other marital status groups. Figure 7.5 describes graphically an analysis of sex differentials by martial status and education for deaths from diseases of the cardiovascular system (excluding cerebrovascular diseases). In Moscow, as in Finland, the sex ratio of deaths differs less by educational level among the married than it does among divorcees; among highly educated divorcees, men are eight times more likely than women to die from cardiovascular diseases compared to four times for divorced men with incomplete secondary education.

Discussion

It has so far been impossible to conduct a detailed validation of the death certificates. However, detailed examination of the data has been undertaken (including analysis of trends by cause of death, study of daily rates and seasonal variations) and no important discontinuities or other evidence of poor data quality have been identified, (Chenet *et al.* 1998a; McKee *et al.* 1998b). The lack of a denominator disaggregated by the socio-economic variables of interest is regrettable but this will not be available in Russia in the foreseeable future. Using a proportional analysis method to overcome this issue is not without shortcomings, but the results presented here are entirely consistent with those presented in another study based on the 1994 Russian micro-census (Shkolnikov *et al.* 1998).

This research confirms the existence of large socio-economic differentials in mortality in the Russian capital. These differentials seem to be even larger than in the west, a finding that tends to be consistent with results from other countries of the former communist bloc (Koupilova *et al.* 1998). It is particularly interesting to note that people engaged in manual occupations have a probability of dying from all causes at least twice as high as people engaged in non-manual occupations, this despite the glorification of industrial labour under the former communist system. Another important finding is the confirmation of research from Hungary and Poland that shows a protective effect of marriage in eastern Europe (Hajdu *et al.* 1995; Watson 1995). However, this protective effect is much stronger for men than for women. Also noteworthy is the particularly poor performance of divorced men: in Russia, alimonies are collected directly from the ex-husband's salary and are fixed at 25 per cent of income for one child, 33 per cent for two children and 50 per cent for three or more children (Valetas 1994). In many ways this ensures greater economic protection for divorced women than in the west (Burkhauser *et al.* 1991; Valetas 1994). Moreover, it is easy to understand how in times of high inflation, divorced men would find themselves with absolutely nothing left to live on. The relative protection of divorced women in Russia also stems from the greater use of the family network: divorced women can easily rely on their parents to look after children. Economic explanations are probably also behind the higher probability of dying experienced by widows.

However, and in contrast to what has been observed in many western European countries (Macintyre and Hunt 1997) these socio-economic differentials seem to be more pronounced among women than among men. This is not only the case for alcohol related mortality or violent deaths, where the smaller numbers of female deaths could give rise to such results, but also for the leading causes of female deaths, that is, cardiovascular and cerebrovascular diseases. Steeper gradients among women for cardiovascular diseases mortality have also been reported in Scotland and Finland (Koskinen and Martelin 1994; Morrison *et al.* 1997).

The particular pattern of the mortality crisis in Russia, with young adults being much more affected than children or elderly people, has led many observers to point to socio-psychological stress as the main factor behind the mortality crisis (Shapiro 1994). There is increasing evidence that the female excess morbidity observed in many western countries is in particular due to women's higher susceptibility to mental health and stress related problems (Verbrugge 1989; Macintyre et al. 1996). Although the link between stress and mortality is not yet totally clear, it would therefore not be surprising to see a female disadvantage in this situation of high social stress. However, this is not the case: female mortality rates have not increased to the same extent as male mortality rates. Moreover, in 1989 (the year of the last census in Russia) women with lower education had a mortality rate from all causes already 60 per cent lower than that of men with higher education, a difference that has widened during the crisis (Shkolnikov et al. 1998). The current research has revealed, however, that women of a lower socio-economic status have been disproportionately affected by the changes.

One of the hypotheses explored repeatedly in the west concerning increasing sex mortality differentials has been that, with increasing equality in society and social roles, men's and women's lifestyles would converge and so would mortality. However, no research seems to have confirmed the convergence hypothesis except maybe for smoking (Koskinen et al. 1995; Nathanson 1995). In Russia, women have been involved in the paid labour market for a long time and still experience a much lower mortality rate than men. Moreover, Russian women still do not smoke much, and even if Muscovites are more likely than the rest of the female Russian population to smoke, it remains relatively rare. Smoking in Russia is also stratified by socio-economic status. Those women who have completed either secondary or vocational education as opposed to tertiary or only primary education are more likely to be current smokers, a distribution that is not consistent with the observed increased in mortality (McKee and Britton 1998). If a high smoking prevalence in Russia could explain the long term high mortality, it is difficult to think of a mechanism that could link smoking and the 1990s mortality crisis.

Alcohol drinking, often associated with stress, is a common feature of Russian life. Indeed, it seems that excess binge drinking has been one of the most important factors of the Russian mortality crisis (Meslé et al. 1994; Leon et al. 1997; Shkolnikov and Nemstov 1997; Chenet et al. 1998b). Not only has alcohol drinking been responsible for the rise in directly alcohol related mortality and accidental and violent deaths but also there is evidence that the Russian pattern of drinking (mostly spirits and in binges) is partly responsible for the rise in cardiovascular mortality (Vikhert *et al.* 1986; McKee and Britton 1998). Research using the same database as the present one shows that mortality from cardio-vascular diseases is higher at weekends, a pattern strikingly similar to deaths due to alcohol poisoning and from accidents and violence (Chenet *et al.* 1998b). However, this association was not statistically significant for women although the same pattern of higher number of cardiovascular and cerebrovascular deaths at weekends was observed.

Given that the socio-economic gradient is steeper for women, then it is understandable that male excess probability of dying is greater among the most privileged segments of society. However, the magnitude of this phenomenon is very surprising, in particular for cardiovascular diseases. However, it is not clear whether this pattern is due to a par-ticular disadvantage of women of lower socio-economic background in Moscow or to a very effective protection of women of a higher status. Vallin (1988, 1996) argues that not only should sex mortality differen-tials be considered in terms of 'bad male behaviour' but also one should take account of the 'virtues' of the female sex. This would fit quite well with the above findings: gender typing is still very pronounced in Russia and, as Lissyutkina puts it:

> Soviet women cannot share the hostility of their Western sisters to the ritualised relationship between men and women. Such gestures as men kissing a woman's hand, and other ways of emphasising a woman's weakness, represent a return to feudal chivalrous culture, that is enthusiastically received by Soviet women.
>
> (Lissyutkina 1993: 274)

The social pressure to behave 'like a lady' might have protected at least some segments of the female population from some of the risk factors most common in Russian society, such as alcohol consumption. In contrast, alcohol drinking is common among men of all social back-grounds. Indeed, some of the success of the Gorbachev anti-alcohol campaign has been linked to his willingness to tackle drinking among the Russian political elite and intelligentsia (Tarschys 1993). This is also indirectly confirmed by the fact that the socio-economic gradients for accidents and violence are so much lower than for directly related alcohol mortality: since abstinence from alcohol is rare in Russian men regard-less of social status, most men are at some increased risk of alcohol related accidents and hence the social differentials are relatively small; sufficiently heavy drinking to precipitate deaths directly attributable to alcohol is, however, more socially stratified (Chenet *et al.* 1998a).

Survey data on the prevalence of risk factors that allow meaning-ful international comparisons between men and women are very rare.

However, the protective effect of feminine gender typing seems to be confirmed by a few studies. Russian men have been reported to drink more, smoke more and have a higher total cholesterol and body mass index than American men, while Russian women drink less, smoke less and have a lower total cholesterol level than American women (Deev *et al.* 1998). Similarly, a survey comparing Finnish and Russian Karelia showed that Russian men smoke more than Finnish men while Russian women smoke less than Finnish women (Laatikainen *et al.* 1999). Finally, a study comparing Finnish and Russian (Moscow) drinking habits also showed that Russian women drink less than Finnish women, drink less often, and get intoxicated less often while the opposite is true for men (Simpura *et al.* 1997).

Conclusion

Sex differentials in mortality in central and eastern Europe are higher than in most countries of the west despite the fact that, before the transition, women were engaged in the labour force to a larger extent than in the west and apparently benefited from an array of measures allowing them to combine family and working life. The excess male mortality is a result of high mortality rates from accidents and violence at younger ages combined with very high rates of degenerative diseases in later life. However, there are marked differences from one country to another as to the particular causes of death. In Russia, it seems that directly and indirectly alcohol related mortality plays a particularly important role.

However, analysis of mortality in Moscow during the mid-1990s shows that for most causes of death, socio-economic differentials are far greater for women than for men. This is of particular concern. Diseases of the circulatory system, accidents and violence, and directly alcohol related mortality are the main causes of deaths behind the Russian mortality crisis of the early 1990s. Although mortality rates have remained lower among women than men, such differentials imply that women of lower social status have suffered disproportionately from the shaky transition to a market economy, confirming early fears that the process of marketization would be particularly harmful for vulnerable social groups and women in particular (Moghadam 1993). Another aspect of these higher female differentials could be that harmful behaviour is far less socially stratified among men than among women, a hypothesis somewhat confirmed as far as alcohol consumption is concerned.

Far more research is needed on socio-economic and gender differentials in central and eastern Europe, research that could also answer some of the questions that have puzzled western researchers for some time. The hypothesis that some intrinsic male disadvantage makes men more vulnerable to adverse social and material conditions (Macintyre 1993) seems to be confirmed by the fact that during the transition towards a market economy, the sex differential in life expectancy at birth increased in all countries of central and eastern Europe. Increased female labour force participation and lower sex mortality differentials definitely do not seem to go together hand in hand thus confirming western findings (Koskinen *et al.* 1995; Nathanson 1995). On the other hand, the higher female socio-economic differentials together with higher male excess probability of dying among the more educated seems to confirm that, as hypothesized by Vallin (1995), the same socio-cultural factors are behind both socio-economic differentials and gender differentials in mortality.

Acknowledgements

This chapter draws on work funded by the UK Department for International Development (DfID). However, DfID can accept no responsibility for the views expressed. Special thanks are due to Seppo Koskinen of the National Public Health Institute, Finland, for his support and comments at an earlier stage of this research.

References

Burkhauser, R., Duncan, G., Hauser, R. and Berntsen, R. (1991) Wife or Frau, women do worse: a comparison of men and women in the United States and Germany after marital dissolution, *Demography*, 28: 353–60.

Charlton, J. (1996) Which areas are healthiest?, *Population Trends*, 83 (Spring): 17–23.

Chenet, L., McKee, M., Fulop, N. *et al.* (1996) Changing life expectancy in central Europe: is there a single reason?, *Journal of Public Health Medicine*, 18: 329–36.

Chenet, L., Leon, D., McKee, M. and Vassin, S. (1998a) Deaths from alcohol and violence in Moscow: socio-economic determinants, *European Journal of Population*, 14: 19–37.

Chenet, L., McKee, M., Leon, D., Shkolnikov, V. and Vassin, S. (1998b) Alcohol and cardiovascular mortality in Moscow: new evidence of a causal association, *Journal of Epidemiology and Community Health*, 52: 772–4.

Deev, A., Shestov, D., Abernathy, J., Kapustina, A., Muhina, N. and Irving, S. (1998) Association of alcohol consumption to mortality in middle-aged U.S. and Russian men and women, *Annals of Epidemiology*, 8: 147–53.

Eisenstein, Z. (1993) Eastern European male democracies: a problem of unequal equalities, in N. Funk and M. Mueller (eds) *Gender Politics and*

Post-communism: Reflections from Eastern Europe and the Former Soviet Union. London: Routledge.

Funk, N. (1993) Women and post-communism, in N. Funk and M. Mueller (eds) *Gender Politics and Post-communism: Reflections from Eastern Europe and the Former Soviet Union.* London: Routledge.

Hajdu, P., McKee, M. and Bojan, F. (1995) Changes in premature mortality differentials by marital status in Hungary and in England and Wales, *European Journal of Public Health*, 5: 559–64.

Heitlinger, A. (1993) The impact of transition communism on the status of women in the Czech and Slovak Republics, in N. Funk and M. Mueller (eds) *Gender Politics and Post-communism: Reflections from Eastern Europe and the Former Soviet Union.* London: Routledge.

Juel, K. and Sjøl, A. (1995) Decline in mortality from heart disease in Denmark: some methodological problems, *Journal of Clinical Epidemiology*, 48: 467–72.

Karro, H., Klimas, V. and Lazdane, G. (1997) Reproductive health in the Baltic countries, *Choice*, 26: 13–17.

Koskinen, S. and Martelin, T. (1994) Pourquoi les femmes sont-elles moins inégales que les hommes devant la mort?, *Population*, 48: 395–414.

Koskinen, S., Martelin, T., Martikainen, P. and Valkonen, T. (1995) Convergence of lifestyle and trends in the sex mortality ratio among the middle aged in Finland, *Yearbook of Population Research in Finland*, 32: 32–44.

Koupilova, I., Vagero, D., Leon, D. A. *et al.* (1998) Social variation in size at birth and preterm delivery in the Czech Republic and Sweden, 1989–91, *Paediatr-Perinat-Epidemiol*, 12: 7–24.

Kozakiewicz, M. (1997) Poland – the struggle for 'free choice' continues, *Choice*, 26: 18–20.

Laatikainen, T., Vartiainen, E. V. and Puska, P. (1999) Smoking and smoking cessation process in the Republic of Karelia, Russia, compared to North Karelia, Finland, *Journal of Epidemiology and Community Health*.

Leon, D., Chenet, L., Shkolnikov, V. *et al.* (1997) Huge variation in Russian mortality rates 1984–1994: artefact, alcohol, or what?, *Lancet*, 350: 383–8.

Lissyutkina, L. (1993) Soviet women at the crossroads of perestroika, in N. Funk and M. Mueller (eds) *Gender Politics and Post-communism: Reflections from Eastern Europe and the Former Soviet Union.* London: Routledge.

McDowall, M. (1983) Adjusting proportional mortality ratios for the influence of extraneous causes of death, *Statistics in Medicine*, 2: 267–475.

Macintyre, S. (1993) Gender differences in longevity and health in Eastern and Western Europe, in S. Platt, H. Thomas, S. Scott and G. Williams (eds) *Locating Health: Sociological and Historical Explanation.* Aldershot: Ashgate.

Macintyre, S. and Hunt, K. (1997) Socio-economic position, gender and health: how do they interact?, *Journal of Health Psychology*, 2(3): 315–34.

Macintyre, S., Hunt, K. and Sweeting, H. (1996) Gender differences in health: are things really as simple as they seem?, *Social Science and Medicine*, 42(4): 617–24.

McKee, M. and Britton, A. (1998) The positive relationship between alcohol and heart disease in Eastern Europe: potential physiological mechanisms, *Journal of Royal Society of Medicine*, 91: 402–7.

McKee, M., Chenet, L., Fulop, N. *et al.* (1996) Explaining the health divide in Germany: contribution of major causes of death to the difference in life expectancy at birth between East and West, *Z. f. Gesundheitswis.*, 4: 214–24.

McKee, M., Bobak, M., Rose, R., Shkolnikov, V., Chenet, L. and Leon, D. (1998a) Patterns of smoking in Russia, *Tobacco Control*, 7: 22–6.

McKee, M., Sanderson, C., Chenet, L., Vassin, S. and Shkolnikov, V. (1998b) Seasonal variation in mortality in Moscow, *Journal of Public Health Medicine*, 20: 268–274.

Meslé, F., Shkolnikov, V. and Vallin, J. (1994) Brusque montée des morts violentes en Russie, *Population*, 49: 780–90.

Meslé, F., Shkolnikov, V., Hertrich, V. and Vallin, J. (1995) Tendance Récentes de la Mortalité par cause en Russie, 1965–1993. Dossiers et Récherche No. 50. Paris: Institut National d'Etudes Demographiques (INED).

Moghadam, V. (1993) Gender dynamics of economic and political change: efficiency, equality, and women, in V. Moghadam (ed.) *Democratic Reform and the Position of Women in Transitional Economies*. Oxford: Clarendon.

Molyneux, M. (1987) Women in socialist societies: problems of theory and practice, in K. Young, C. Wolkowitz and R. McCullagh (eds) *Of Marriage and the Market: Women's Subordination Internationally and its Lessons*. London: Routledge.

Morrison, C., Woodward, M., Leslie, W. and Tunstall-Pedoe, H. (1997) Effect of socio-economic group on incidence of, management of, and survival after myocardial infarction and coronary death: analysis of a community coronary event register, *British Medical Journal*, 314: 541–6.

Nathanson, C. (1995) Mortality and the position of women in developed countries, in A. Lopez, G. Caselli and T. Valkonen (eds) *Adult Mortality in Developed Countries: From Description to Explanation*. Oxford: Clarendon.

Nickel, H. (1993) Women in the German Democratic Republic and in the New Federal States: looking backward and forward (five theses), in N. Funk and M. Mueller (eds) *Gender Politics and Post-communism: Reflections from Eastern Europe and the Former Soviet Union*. London: Routledge.

Nowicka, W. (1995) The fight for reproductive rights in Central and Eastern Europe. Poland: Catholic backlash, *Planned Parenthood Challenges*, 2: 23–4.

Ortner, S. (1974) Is female to male as nature is to culture, in M. Rosaldo and L. Lamphere (eds) *Women, Culture and Society*. Stanford, CA: Stanford University Press.

Pollard, J. (1982) The expectation of life and its relationship to mortality, *Journal of the Institute of Actuaries*, 9: 225–40.

Pollard, J. (1987) Cause of death and expectation of life: some international comparisons, in J. Vallin, S. D'Souza and A. Palloni (eds) *Measurement of Mortality: New Approaches*. Liège: Oxford University Press.

Ryan, M. (1995) Alcoholism and rising mortality in the Russian Federation, *British Medical Journal*, 310: 646–8.

Shapiro, J. (1994) *The Russian Mortality Crisis and its Causes*, working paper no. 99. Stockholm: Östekonomiska Institutet.

Shkolnikov, V. and Nemstov, A. (1997) The anti-alcohol campaign and variations in Russian mortality, in J. Bobadilla, C. Costello and F. Mitchell (eds) *Premature Death in the New Independent States*. Washington, DC: National Academy Press.

Shkolnikov, V., Leon, D., Adamets, S., Andreev, E. and Deev, A. (1998) Educational level and adult mortality in Russia: an analysis of routine data 1979–1994, *Social Science and Medicine*, 47(3): 357–69.

Simpura, J., Levin, B. and Mustonen, H. (1997) Russian drinking in the 1990s: patterns and trends in international comparisons, in J. Simpura and B. Levin (eds) *Demystifying Russian Drinking*. Saarijärvi: Gummerus Kirjapaino Oy.

Tarschys, D. (1993) The success of a failure: Gorbachev's alcohol policy 1985–88, *Europe-Asia Studies*, 45: 7–25.

Valetas, M. (1994) Le paiement des pensions alimentaires en France et en Russie, *Population*, 49: 451–71.

Vallin, J. (1988) *Evolution sociale et baisse de la mortalité: conquête ou reconquête d'un avantage féminin*, Dossier et recherche no. 17. Paris: INED.

Vallin, J. (1995) Can sex differentials in mortality be explained by socio-economic mortality differentials?, in A. Lopez, G. Caselli and T. Valkonen (eds) *Adult Mortality in Developed Countries: From Description to Explanation*. Oxford: Clarendon.

Vallin, J. (1996) Les differences de mortalité entre sexes, in *Demography: Analysis and Synthesis*, Conference proceedings vol. 3. Siena: Certosa di Pontignano.

Varvasovszky, Z. and McKee, M. (1998) Alcohol policy in Hungary, *Addiction*, 93(12): 1815–28.

Varvasovszky, Z., Bain, C. and McKee, M. (1997) Deaths from cirrhosis in Poland and Hungary: the impact of different alcohol policies during the 1980s, *Journal of Epidemiology and Community Health*, 51: 197–71.

Verbrugge, L. (1989) The twain meet: empirical evidence of sex differences in health and mortality, *Journal of Health and Social Behavior*, 20 (September): 282–304.

Vikhert, A., Tsiplenkova, V. and Cherpachenko, N. (1986) Alcohol cardiomyopathy and sudden cardiac death, *Journal of the American College of Cardiology*, 8: 3A–11A.

Watson, P. (1995) Explaining rising mortality among men in Eastern Europe, *Social Science and Medicine*, 41(7): 923–34.

Wolchik, S. (1993) Women and the politics of transition in Central and Eastern Europe, in V. Moghadam (ed.) *Democratic Reforms and the Position of Women in Transitional Economies*. Oxford: Clarendon.

Index